TORE GODAL AND THE EVOLUTION OF GLOBAL HEALTH

I0054512

This book is an interconnected history of the evolution of global health in the decades before 2019, told through the prism of six decisive moments in which individuals from the World Health Organization (WHO), philanthropic foundations, academia and bilateral agencies came together to shape the world.

These critical junctures are accessed via the life and work of Norwegian immunologist Tore Godal, one of the most influential health physicians of all time. Godal's career over the past 50 years offers a window into the profound events that have shaped the health and well-being of millions across the globe, including the first free donation of a drug for the treatment of river blindness; the entry of the Bill and Melinda Gates Foundation into the global health arena with a $750 million start-up grant for GAVI, the Global Alliance for Vaccines and Immunization; the 50% reduction in under-five mortality rates this century; the emergence of insecticide bed nets as the cornerstone of WHO malaria control; the rise of maternal and child health on the global political agenda; and the connection between Ebola and the creation of the Coalition for Epidemic Preparedness Innovations (CEPI) in 2017.

Exploring the ways in which the trajectory of global health has interwoven with the rich life and legacy of Godal, this book is a crucial resource for any reader interested in global health.

Conrad Keating is the Writer-in-Residence and Visiting Professor at the School of Medicine, Trinity College Dublin. He works on the social history of medicine and the history of science and was previously the Writer-in-Residence at the Wellcome Unit for the History of Medicine at the University of Oxford. His most recent publication is the widely acclaimed *Anthony Cerami: A Life in Translational Medicine* (2021). Previous work includes *Kenneth Warren and the Great Neglected Diseases of Mankind Programme: The Transformation of Geographical Medicine in the US and Beyond* (2017); *Great Medical Discoveries: An Oxford Story* (2013); and *Smoking Kills: The Revolutionary Life of Richard Doll* (2009). Keating has an ongoing ten-part *Art of Medicine* essay series on the history of randomised controlled trials in *The Lancet*.

Routledge Studies in the History of Science, Technology and Medicine

For more information about this series, please visit: www.routledge.com/Routledge-Studies-in-the-History-of-Science-Technology-and-Medicine/book-series/HISTSCI

Tore Godal and the Evolution of Global Health

Conrad Keating

Routledge
Taylor & Francis Group

NEW YORK AND LONDON

First published 2024
by Routledge
605 Third Avenue, New York, NY 10158

and by Routledge
4 Park Square, Milton Park, Abingdon, Oxon, OX14 4RN

Routledge is an imprint of the Taylor & Francis Group, an informa business

© 2024 Conrad Keating

The right of Conrad Keating to be identified as author of this work has
been asserted in accordance with sections 77 and 78 of the Copyright,
Designs and Patents Act 1988.

All rights reserved. No part of this book may be reprinted or reproduced
or utilised in any form or by any electronic, mechanical, or other means,
now known or hereafter invented, including photocopying and recording,
or in any information storage or retrieval system, without permission in
writing from the publishers.

Trademark notice: Product or corporate names may be trademarks
or registered trademarks, and are used only for identification and
explanation without intent to infringe.

ISBN: 978-1-032-42698-3 (hbk)
ISBN: 978-1-032-42700-3 (pbk)
ISBN: 978-1-003-36385-9 (ebk)

DOI: 10.4324/9781003363859

Contents

Acknowledgements

Writing a book about the decisive moments in global health has been an extraordinary experience given that it occurred as a global pandemic unfolded that shook the foundations of human life. There can be no more poignant reminder of why we should all care about global health than the events of recent years as communities around the world collectively grappled with the COVID-19 pandemic on multiple personal and societal levels. Until this point, one of the reasons why global health had not been paramount in most people's minds, particularly in the global north, is because this is a field dominated by science. It is after all the business of creating vaccines, of thinking about immunisation strategies and of identifying pathogens. This was often seen as an abstract, inaccessible world, divorced from the practical realities and vocabularies of everyday life. This is very clearly no longer the case. This book in many ways is an introduction to a subject with which we are all, for better or worse, inextricably associated: it tells the story of the emergence of global health as a field of scientific, political and economic activity. This is an interconnected history that uses the life of the immunologist and global health leader, Tore Godal, as a common thread linking key 'moments' in the development of global health thinking and action.

I'm certainly not alone in thinking that storytelling is a very important contributing – some think essential – element to the public understanding of medicine and biomedical research. We are after all creatures of story, and this is how we make sense of the world. Consequently, I owe a debt of gratitude to Trinity College Dublin for their farsightedness in allowing me access to my office to write this book once the most restrictive quarantine measures eased. How strange and almost incomprehensible it was to walk through the completely uninhabited campus, and to see Parliament Square devoid of the hum of human activity.

My profound thanks goes to two people without whom this volume would not exist. First to Tore Godal, because this book is an act of synthesis, a fusion of our collective endeavour and a product of his intellectual generosity. Second, my research was funded by the inimitable President of the Gender Equality Division and Director of Vaccine Development, Global Health Surveillance, Diarrhoea and Enteric Diseases at the Bill & Melinda Gates Foundation, Anita Zaidi. Dr

Zaidi's vision, support and encouragement were constants throughout the writing process.

For their principled interventions in my thinking and global health education, I'm immensely grateful to Richard Peto, Jeremy Farrar, Bridget Ogilvie, Dean Jamison, Gus Nossal, Tim Evans, Joe Cook, Steve Meshnick, Tony Cerami, Peter Smith, Brian Greenwood, Chris Murray, David Bradley, Bill Foege, David Heymann, Richard Horton, Seth Berkley, Carol Bellamy, Stanley Plotkin, Gro Harlem Brundtland, Alan Lopez, Chris Elias, Barry Bloom, Bill Campbell, Don Bundy, Adrian Hopkins, Bjorn Tylefors, Uche Amazigo, Daniel Boakye, Hans Remme, Simon Bush, Adrian Hopkins, Ripley Ballou, Steve Lindsay, Helga Fogstad, Rajiv Shah and Peter Piot.

Additionally, for their invaluable perspectives on the political realities and everyday workings of global health institutions, I am indebted to the cooperation and trust of Amie Batson, Bo Stenson, Lisa Jacobs, Jens Stoltenberg, Viroj Tangcharoensathien, Alice Albright, Paul Fife, Violaine Mitchell, Kathy Calvin, Morten Wetland, Jonas Ghar Støre, Bard Vegar Solhjell, Monique Vledder, Suprotik Basu, Lene Jeanette Lothe, Robert Orr, Amina Mohammed, Ariel Pablos-Mendez, Marie-Paule Kieny, John-Arne Røttingen, Mark Feinberg, Børge Brende, Swati Gupta, Bjørn Myrvang, Andy Crump, David Evans, Sue Tyrrell and Tarald Brautaset.

I would like to thank all my colleagues in the School of Medicine, in particular, Michael Gill, Martina Hennessy, Brian Lawlor, and my close friends in Old Anatomy, Siobhan Ward, Philomena McAteer and Barry Lyons.

Of course, every good book needs a skilled editor, and I've been very fortunate in being able to work so constructively with the superb Max Novick at Routledge, and both he and his editorial team deserve special thanks for their assiduous work and attention to detail.

My last and deepest thanks are to Jen, for her love, literary advice, wise counsel and who repeatedly laid aside her own work to answer my queries or to read drafts of this book. She has been entirely unselfish and generous with her insightful brilliance and stylistic gifts. Not a day goes by when I'm not blissfully conscious that Jen is the most important person in my universe, and her presence gives my life an air of freedom.

Conrad Keating,
Trinity College Dublin, August 2022

Introduction

Decisive Moments in Global Health and the Life of a Medical Scientist

It is better to go skiing and think of God, than go to church and think of sport.

Fridtjof Nansen

When I first began to visualise this book in the early months of 2018, my intention was to take the reader into the fascinating, multidimensional world of what had previously been called 'international health' or 'tropical medicine' and increasingly since the beginning of this century, 'global health'. In very broad terms, the latter deals with the health of populations in a worldwide context, focusing not simply on improving the quality of health in communities across the globe, but also in foregrounding issues of health equity, particularly in the global south. The field 'emphasises transnational health issues, determinants, and solutions; involves many disciplines within and beyond the health sciences and promotes interdisciplinary collaboration; and is a synthesis of population-based prevention with individual-level clinical care'.[1] Perhaps without many beyond the immediate field itself realising, global health has in recent years become one of the pre-eminent areas not just of medical research but also of foreign policy, philanthropy, finance and international cooperation.

My aim was always to write for both the general reader and the academic community, but how would I be able to explain to that audience in a clear, understandable and entertaining way the complex, scientised world of global health, a world defined by questions about immunology; about how vaccines work against a highly infectious disease; or indeed the intricacies of translational research, molecular medicine, or recombinant technologies; and the indispensable role of B cells and T cells in preventing disease and promoting human health? I needn't have worried; the chaos and devastation caused by the COVID-19 pandemic marked a catastrophic inflection point in modern human history. SARS-CoV-2, first officially recognised in China in December 2019, made everyone instantaneously aware of the concept and fragility of 'global health', while the ensuing process of understanding, treating and preventing the disease helped to create a common vocabulary across the world, enabling everyday considerations of

DOI: 10.4324/9781003363859-1

such previously esoteric subjects as 'randomised placebo-controlled trials', and the 'utility of anti-SARS-CoV-2 monoclonal antibodies'. My book, however, does not address the COVID-19 pandemic directly, although myriad admirable publications have, and will, tell how this story is one of the outstanding scientific achievements of our age, and how it took only 11 months from the publication of the pathogen's gene sequence to the development of several effective vaccines against the disease.[2]

By ending where the COVID-19 pandemic begins, this study examines the evolution of global health through the exploration of six 'decisive moments' in which assemblages of people from the World Health Organization, philanthropic foundations, academia, bilateral agencies or other institutions came together to shape the world that we now inhabit. This conceptual framework acts as a template that progressively introduces the reader to these formative evidence-based interventions that have greatly improved human health, setting biomedical science in the broader contexts of politics, economics and social justice. The advantage of this approach, in contrast to meticulously studying a singular episode, such as the eradication of smallpox, the discovery of penicillin or the 1918 influenza pandemic, is that it becomes possible to gradually identify and expose the often invisible architectures – human, intellectual and financial – that underpin the vast field of global health. In turn, this begins to bring added dimensions into view, not least by revealing how one individual global health challenge is not only about that specific undertaking, but has an implicit interconnection in shaping the intellectual and practical bedrock of another. For example, the final chapter of this volume looks at the development of the Coalition for Epidemic Preparedness Innovations (CEPI), established in 2017, as a mechanism of preparing in advance for the pandemics that have intermittently occurred throughout human history. This thematic chapter uses the Ebola virus disease epidemic, which broke out in West Africa in December 2013, as a presentiment of the COVID-19 pandemic; tellingly many of the individuals, pharmaceutical companies, and even countries and philanthropic bodies that were involved in the efforts to control the Ebola epidemic were also key actors in the planning, financing, and design of CEPI. Clearly, ideas have a genealogy, and the coming together of various assemblages over the past 50 years can be identified as 'decisive moments' in the continuous and principled attempts to reduce human suffering and to improve global public health. In other words, the decisive moments explored in this volume are decisive precisely because they were not only formative episodes in the containment of Ebola or in the reduction of infant mortality, but also because they were critical junctures in the emergence of new ideas, strategies and priorities that have shaped the over-arching global health agenda. For the reader, this analytical device of describing 'moments' that became pivotal in the life of the global health idea may well resonate and draw parallels with the decisive events that have influenced the cadence and direction of their own lives.

How then might one narrow one's scope to condense the rich world of global health into a text-based project? What unifying thread can help to stitch together health-based interventions across many different parts of the world? This book uses the life of one man, the Norwegian immunologist and leading global health activist, Tore Godal, to access this far broader, complex global history. Godal, described by *The Lancet* in 2019 as the 'quiet colossus of global health', is one of the most influential global health physicians of all time.[3] In contrast to some other influential global health leaders,[4] Godal does not have a reputation for making electrifying conference speeches or being hyperbolic; he is unassuming, laconic and quietly spoken, while at the same time being self-confident, compellingly persuasive and unrelenting in pursuit of what he believes will advance human health. His remarkable scientific career extends across six decades and offers a window onto decisive moments that have influenced the health and well-being of millions across the globe, encompassing the first free donation of a drug by the pharmaceutical giant Merck for the treatment of river blindness; the World Bank's decision that health should be calculated as an investment and not an expenditure; the entry of The Bill and Melinda Gates Foundation into the global health arena via a $750 million start-up grant for GAVI (the Global Alliance for Vaccines and Immunization); the Roll Back Malaria campaign; and the pioneering work to avert an Ebola pandemic in 2014–2015. Featuring comprehensive oral testimony from Godal and other key individuals, the book illustrates the fascinating chemistry of having the right people, in the right place, at the right time. This is a story relevant to everyone on the planet, and one that has never been told on such a coherent, human and understandable scale. By exploring the ways in which the trajectory of global health over the past decades has interwoven with the rich life and legacy of Godal, the following chapters jettison the standard linear life narrative in favour of spotlighting pivotal moments, while retaining for the reader the human connective tissue that links the personal and the global. Consequently, this book is not an absolute biography of Tore Godal, nor is it a comprehensive history of global health. In fact, there remain many episodes and important moments in the latter that deserve exploration in their own right. Rather, the following pages bring us into Godal's world and, in doing so, bring us to the very heart of what global health has become. This is in some ways a question of how to explore complex topics at scale: understanding the man allows us to begin to understand the wider field.

In this sense, using one individual's professional life as a lens allows us to embark on a journey that explores the workings of global institutions such as the World Health Organiation, taking us to the heart of scientific efforts to treat leprosy, to prevent the Ebola outbreak from becoming a pandemic, and to high-level initiatives within global finance and philanthropy. In doing so, we travel from the offices of the World Bank in Washington; to the World Health Organization in Geneva; to government departments, pharmaceutical companies and private individuals on five continents; to villages, fields and laboratories stretching from

Ghana and Ethiopia to Bangladesh and Vietnam. Crucially, this is not a story told from above or below, but from within, offering breadth of experience between the global north and south, and one that feeds into growing curiosity in international politics, medicine, education, and civil society about how world-changing initiatives do (or don't work), how ideas are born and translated, and how future action in the pursuit of health and income equity around the globe can be sustained. These diverse episodes are woven together through Godal's own life, and generate not simply a sense of one of the most influential physicians of our time, but more importantly, insights into the vibrant world of global health; one that has transformed, and continues to transform, the lives of millions of people.

In the opinion of the world-renowned health economist Chris Murray, 'Tore was not only present in many of the critical moments in global health; he has been instrumental in making them happen'.[5] From the outset, whether through direct participation, campaigning zeal or convening power, Godal's track record is impressive. After conducting pioneering work into the treatment of leprosy in Ethiopia, in 1986 Godal became Director of the UN-based Special Programme for Research and Training in Tropical Diseases (TDR for short), where he helped to transform our understanding of disease. He directed research programmes showing the effectiveness of the drug ivermectin in treating river blindness and supported studies which showed that the most efficient method of distributing the drug at scale across vast areas of Africa was via community-directed treatment. In the early 1990s, dismayed by WHO's ambiguous position on bed nets for malaria prevention, Godal took a calculated risk and put all of TDR's malaria field budget into large-scale randomised controlled trials, which showed how insecticide-treated bed nets could drastically reduce malaria mortality. Today, insecticide-treated bed nets form the cornerstone of the WHO's Global Malaria Control Programme. Godal's decade as Director of TDR became synonymous with two discernible features: first, he was seen as someone who was serious about using science to improve the health of communities in emerging economies; and second, his tenure served as a model for enabling WHO to shed its aversion to working with the private sector.

Following his enforced retirement at the age of 60, in 1999 Godal then headed the Working Group that planned the development of GAVI, the Vaccine Alliance, supported by a grant of US$750 million from Bill Gates. The donation, unprecedented in its magnitude, led to Godal becoming GAVI's first CEO in 2000. One of the great global health success stories this century has been the halving of under-five mortality, and today, GAVI has vaccinated more than three-quarters of a billion children and saved 13 million lives.[6] Several years later, in 2005, Tore Godal found another new alchemising role when he became a special adviser to Norway's then Prime Minister, Jens Stoltenberg, and helped to elevate Norway into the highest echelons of global health power and prestige. Acting almost 'as an arm of the Norwegian government',[7] Godal persuaded Stoltenberg to spend billions of dollars on global health programmes, drawing on his nuanced understanding that politicians need simple persuasive messages that are easily understood by their tax-paying electorate. Consequently, cost-effectiveness was a political and moral imperative for all the global health policies that Godal championed. In his advocacy of cost-effective, life-saving investments, he signposted Stoltenberg and his government to embrace two of the most neglected Millennium Development Goals and, in doing so, reconfigured the outcomes of maternal and child health, particularly in Africa and India. 'Tore convinced me', Stoltenberg magnanimously declared in 2019,

> and the whole of Norway that we should become the lead nation for child health and vaccines. No-one else could have convinced me to spend billions on child health and maternal care. Tore Godal is the most expensive Norwegian in history, and the money has been very well spent.[8]

Throughout our recent history, some of the greatest achievements in health have come from extending the reach of scientific and technological breakthroughs

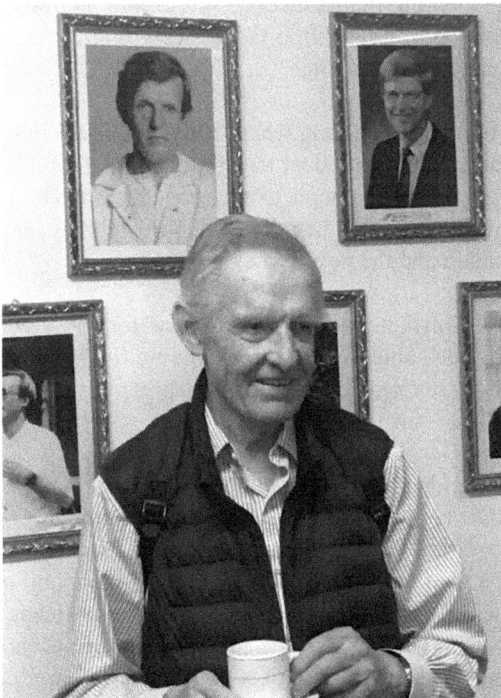

Figure 0.1 Tore Godal in front of a portrait of his younger self at the Armauer Hansen Research Institute, Addis Ababa, Ethiopia, 2018.

Source: Courtesy of Frederik Kristensen/CEPI.

to those populations, who for political and economic reasons were denied their use.[9] Finding efficient and politically realistic ways to spread transformative scientific advances that are in everyday use in the wealthiest countries to the poorest parts of the world where the disease burden is greatest has been, and continues to be, one of Godal's overriding missions. Acting as 'a builder'[10] as he redesigns the architecture of global health, his contribution has been to identify long-standing obstacles and then to bring collections of people and their institutions together to collaborate and make those problems soluble. As we shall see, sometimes this required creating a new institution like GAVI or CEPI, while on other occasions it was more about leveraging existing institutions, as in the case of developing the Global Financing Facility within the World Bank.[11] One of Godal's recognised skills is his ability to conceive and launch new global health ideas and institutions, to safeguard them through the difficult early stages of life to become successful, and then to take a step back, vacating control and kudos and allowing others to take centre stage. This was achieved by a combination of being a kind and 'unassuming'[12] role model, coupled with a real depth of expertise and technical knowledge across both institutional and scientific fields. Godal's intellectual honesty, moral seriousness and complete lack of self-importance, according to the President of the Rockefeller Foundation, Rajiv Shah,

> enabled Tore to create a culture, where people believed in him and his mission. He has an exceptional talent to set a big goal, mobilise people against that goal and somehow get people to be more tethered to him and his mission than to their institutions, and their own job. Tore did it by his moral authority, with determination and the power of example.[13]

So, what exactly constitutes a 'decisive moment' for Tore Godal, the visionary physician who has been able to influence the future of global health by creating durable interventions to elegantly overcome various political, scientific and economic obstacles? In his own words,

> the first step is to identify an important problem that is not being addressed. Secondly, it must be technically feasible and scientifically based, if not, then [the project] must build a scientific base. Thirdly, I had to have a sense that it would mobilise political interest, and the potential to mobilise finance. . . . A decisive moment is in some respects like when a virus leaps from an animal to a human being. Then as it starts to spread, it adapts through mutations to human beings and transmission between them becomes easier. Similarly, adaptions take place in projects or initiatives that represent smaller decisive moments, until it reaches a kind of steady state. During that phase, getting the right constellation of people involved is critical.[14]

Using this template, for many decades Godal has helped to stimulate the global health agenda by making research programmes relevant for decision-making in political forums. However, there are many examples of how medical discoveries have become mired in obfuscation,[15] resulting in the loss of millions of lives, as a direct result of evidence-based health research hitting the buffers of the non-evidence-based political world, and the dynamics of how and why individuals and institutions make decisions. Godal's low-key style and inclination to give stage presence to others disguise the fact that he is a politically-savvy, operational guru, who is more interested in getting the right things done in global health, than emphasising who did them. This perhaps goes some way towards explaining why Tore Godal's name remains relatively anonymous to the outside world but not to other global health scientists dedicated to melding biomedical science and political will to create a safer, fairer world. Jeremy Farrar is Director of the Wellcome Trust, Europe's largest medical charity and one of the co-founders with Godal of CEPI.

Tore is a survivor, and he understands the soft dark arts of political influence probably better than anybody else. Tore has been lucky, but you make your own luck, and he has been in a country that is really committed to the global good. Norway stands out as being extraordinary, but that doesn't happen by chance. That happens because of people like Tore.[16]

Chris Elias, meanwhile, is the president of the Global Development Division at the Bill and Melinda Gates Foundation, and he too has witnessed at first hand Godal's ability to bring people and institutions together to solve problems.

Tore has been at the start of so many important initiatives. Most notably for the foundation, he was the first executive director of GAVI. We often say, 'GAVI was one of our first, largest and best investments'. In the very beginning, the foundation made a $750 million commitment, and if you add it all up GAVI is still our largest single investment over twenty something years now. The foundation still invests north of $300 million a year in GAVI, so if you add it all up, Tore has been an expensive friend.[17]

To Dean Jamison, the US economist and lead author of the lodestar publication *World Development Report 1993: Investing in Health*, his relationship with Godal is based on mutual respect.

There are two or three people in the world who when they ask me to do something I do it. And Tore is one of them. Partly that is out of respect and partly affection. And out of a sense that we are very much on the same page in terms of what we are trying to advance in the world. He has been influential in my life.[18]

To his friend, the former prime minister of Norway Jens Stoltenberg, Godal's contribution to global health is historically poignant and occupies the highest national acknowledgement. 'Tore's efforts to help poor people to better health must not be underestimated. He is surely, after Fridtjof Nansen the Norwegian who has saved most lives in the world'.[19] This book is a history of some of the decisive moments in the evolution of global health composed in a rich personal setting.

Notes

1. J. Koplan et al., "Towards a common definition of global health", *The Lancet*, 6 June 2009, 373 (9679), pp. 1993–1995. For more on this vast field and its definition, see R. Beaglehole, R. Bonita, "What is global health?", *Global Health Action*, 2010, 3, 10.3402/gha.v3i0.5142; R. Packard, *A History of Global Health: Interventions Into the Lives of Other Peoples* (Baltimore: Johns Hopkins University Press, 2016).
2. On the Covid pandemic, see, for instance, J. Farrar, A. Ahuja, *Spike: The Virus vs the People, the Inside Story* (London: Profile Books, 2021); R. Horton, *The Covid-19 Catastrophe: What's Gone Wrong and How to Stop It Happening Again* (Cambridge: Polity Press, 2021).
3. R. Lane, "Tore Godal: Quiet colossus of global health", *Lancet*, December 2019, 394, p. 2143.
4. Unlike, for instance, the figure of Ken Warren, Godal's opposite number at the Rockefeller Foundation: C. Keating, *Kenneth Warren and the Great Neglected Diseases of Mankind Programme: The Transformation of Geographical Medicine in the US and Beyond* (New York: Springer, 2017).
5. Interview with Christopher Murray, March 2019.
6. Interview with Seth Berkley, November 2019.
7. Interview with Peter Smith, December 2019.
8. Interview with Jens Stoltenberg, April 2019.
9. R. Shah, "Breakthroughs for development", *Science*, 2011, 333, p. 385.
10. Interview with Jane Halton, December 2021.
11. Interview with Chris Elias, November 2021.
12. Interview with Alan Lopez, August 2020.
13. Interview with Rajiv Shah, January 2022.
14. Interview with Tore Godal, January 2022.
15. An unfortunate example of this phenomenon is Artesunate (an artemisinin derivative), the first-line drug for treatment of severe malaria in the United States. Following the scientific research proving the efficacy of the drug, it was to take 10 to 15 years before the drug was widely used. Because of this delay, probably one million people lost their lives.
16. Interview with Jeremy Farrar, August 2018.
17. Interview with Chris Elias, December 2021.
18. Interview with Dean Jamison, October 2020.
19. Interview with Jens Stoltenberg, April 2019.

1 The Special Programme for Research and Training in Tropical Diseases (TDR)

A spider conducts operations that resemble those of a weaver, and a bee puts to shame many an architect in the construction of her cells. But what distinguishes the worst architect from the best of bees is this, that the architect raises his structure in imagination before he erects it in reality.[1]

Karl Marx

Early Experiences and the Primacy of Storytelling

In 1967, on a bright, green June morning, Tore Godal walked purposefully in the direction of Gamle Festsal, one of the historic main halls of the University of Oslo, where he was going to defend his PhD thesis.[2] The day had added significance for the 28-year doctoral candidate; it coincided with the end of his medical degree. He was about to embark on a career in medicine, and his ambition was to become a District Medical Officer and improve the health and well-being of the people in his home valley in rural Norway.[3] One of his PhD reviewers that morning was Professor Morten Harboe, the leading exponent of modern immunology in Norway, and who subsequently became an expert on the immunology of tuberculosis and leprosy. During the course of the review, Professor Harboe mentioned, rather matter-of-factly, that a few months earlier, he had been invited to establish a leprosy research laboratory in Addis Ababa, Ethiopia. The distinguished immunologist then proceeded to throw Godal's best-laid career plans into disarray, with an astonishing revelation, 'However, I will only take up the post, if you agree to succeed me as director!'[4] At the time, there was no discernible career path for immunologists in tropical disease research, and a colleague of Morten Harboe warned Godal that if he did decide to take up the offer, 'then you can say farewell to an attractive medical career in Norway'.[5] Even in his wildest fantasies, Godal had never imagined being a medical researcher in Africa, but the description of life as a research scientist at the fledgling Armauer Hansen Research Institute in Addis Ababa seemed so otherworldly that it stirred his sense of adventure.

DOI: 10.4324/9781003363859-2

It is fair to say that Godal has always inhabited grand dreams, a product of his childhood and the influence of his mother's ethereal fairy tales of audacity and daring. These stories were often connected to people in distant geographies, and gave a window on life to the young Tore that allowed him to see beyond his own valley home in Western Norway and imagine far-off destinations where dreams could become reality. His mother, Randi Fætten Bojer Godal, was a school-teacher by profession, and her fables of wonder and mythology carried within them metaphors of earthy practicality,[6] with the values of responsibility and use-fulness allied to feelings of belonging. The power of storytelling to infuse the ideals of adventure and daring was reinforced by the mesmerising presence of his maternal grandfather, Johan Bojer (1872–1959), the highly successful novel-ist and dramatist. Bojer, who was brought up in abject poverty, had to triumph over considerable adversity, and was nominated four times for the Nobel Prize in literature.[7] His powerful novels reflected the zeitgeist, winning wide critical acclaim in Norway and beyond. The novel, *The Last of the Vikings* – later pub-lished in English – depicts the harsh lives of resourceful fishermen who spend the winter fishing within the Arctic Circle, in the far north of Norway. Today, he is best known for the social-realistic novel *The Emigrants*, which describes the sacrifices and achievements of the Norwegians that emigrated to the Great Plains of North Dakota in the first quarter of the twentieth century. Bojer also wrote fairy tales that he had learned from his stepmother and then retold them in a dramatically evocative style to Tore and his other grandchildren.

The mysterious intensity of childhood was, for the English poet William Wordsworth, all-important in informing the trajectory and hinterland of later life, and in his poem *My Heart Leaps Up* he describes the child as 'father of the man' and expresses the hope that the wonder present in the childhood gaze could remain intact through adulthood.[8]

> *My heart leaps up when I behold*
> *A rainbow in the sky:*
> *So was it when my life began;*
> *So it is now I am a man;*
> *So be it when I shall grow old,*
> *Or let me die!*
> *The Child is father of the Man;*
> *And I could wish my days to be*
> *Bound each to each by natural piety*

The 'natural piety' allusion, so critical to Wordsworth's romantic understanding of nature, also represented a formative spiritual symbolism in Tore's childhood – his father, Odd Godal, was a Lutheran parish priest in the mountain village of Rauland. From his father, Tore learned the value of stoicism to give perspective and to control the choices he made in life. During these early formative years, he gained the facility to rise above criticism, to embrace a protestant work ethic and to recognise that with righteousness on their side, people can change the world. However, this ethical preparation came at great personal cost, as life in Rauland was far from an Arcadian idyll. Tore Godal was born on 19 May 1939; less than one year later, on 9 April 1940, German forces invaded neutral Norway. The continuous Nazi occupation of the country lasted until the surrender of Germany on 8 May 1945 – the intervening years were divisive, bitter and left painful societal scars.[9] The chaos of World War II cast a shadow over life, and none of Norway's institutions was resistant to its insidious reach. Odd Godal was part of the Resistance movement, and in 1943, gave shelter to the Norwegian commandos who sabotaged the production of heavy water at a hydroelectric power station in Telemark, which Germany needed for the development of nuclear weapons. Although only four years old at the time, Tore recalled the occasion with familial analytical clarity, 'It was the only time my father lied to me. He told me that they were bringing food supplies to distribute around the local town'. Fascism and division were disrupting forces on the pews of his father's church. The traditional nature of rural life in 1940s Norway played out along gender lines within the church congregation, with women occupying benches on one side of the isle, and men the other. However, the five years of war had brought added subdivisions within the parishioners. The churchgoers were segregated further into three distinct political divisions: the true Nazis, the collaborators and members of the resistance movement. The obvious tensions within the congregation took a toll on Odd Godal who felt spiritually conflicted and as a result in 1946 the family left for a new parish in the Eastern part of Norway where Odd would not know the social divisions created by the war. This experience failed to diminish Odd Godal's sense of optimism; he continued to find ways to engage with society, and there was a discernible handing on of social values and a 'can-do spirit' by Odd, and Randi Fætten, to Tore and his two brothers and sister.

These mores and the primary familial experiences absorbed by Godal early in his life had a lasting influence on his interpretation of, and curiosity for, the world around him. As did other, more osmotically embraced patterns of thinking, most notably what Scandinavian's collectively term, '*Janteloven*', or The Law of Jante – the principles and values that culturally guide an individual to live a harmonious and happy life. These were first articulated – but recognised to have antecedents in the nineteenth century – in the form of ten rules in the 1933 satirical novel *The Fugitive Crosses His Tracks* by Askel Sandemose. In the book, the eponymous fictional town of Jante is governed by ten sociological rules that frown on individual success and boastfulness and emphasize adherence to the wider collective. Rule number four perfectly crystallises the ethos of Janteloven: 'You are not to imagine yourself better than *we* are'. In the language of modern life, over-aggrandising or the 'bigging-up', of oneself is seen as vulgar and rude, while the values of equity and fairness are lionised. To a greater or lesser degree, post-war Norwegian (and wider Scandinavian) society evolved immersed in the mind-set of Jantaloven: a stoicism of getting on with daily life, that *you* as an individual are not anything special and that it is possible to have a strong inner self-confident, while at the same time being humble.[10] In 1967, when Professor Morten Harboe offered Tore Godal the opportunity to succeed him as the director of the Armauer Hansen Research Institute (AHRI) in Addis Ababa, he did so in the knowledge that he had found a colleague who was spiritually adventurous, scientifically adept and free of pretension.

The Immunology of Leprosy

Before leaving for Africa, Godal spent 18 months following a peripatetic training programme in Norway and further afield, curated by Morten Harboe, designed to expose him to some of the recent developments in the science of the new immunology. The specialist training included a hospital internship in Tromsø, a city in the Arctic Circle, pathology research at Bergen's Gade Institute, and a nine-month laboratory research course working at the cutting edge of immunology at the National Institute of Medical Research, Mill Hill, London.

The 1950s and 1960s had been exciting decades of discovery in immunology and had laid the foundations for the field to become a dominant force in biomedical science. In 1960, the Australian virologist Frank Macfarlane Burnet and the UK biologist Peter Medawar received the Nobel Prize 'for their discovery of acquired immunological tolerance'.[11] The 'new immunology', as Burnet termed it, of the modern era identified three principal areas of enquiry: the biology of self-recognition, the molecular basis of information transfer and the immunological response in terms of lymphatic cells. At around the same time, the immunologist, James Gowans, a colleague of Medawar, working at the Sir William Dunn School of Pathology, in Oxford showed that 'the mysterious lymphocyte'[12] were not short-lived but circulated between blood and tissue and therefore could patrol the body.[13] Although the lymphocyte is a small and unprepossessing looking white blood cell, Gowans proved that it was the seat of immunological reaction. Building on Gowans' immunologic finding, scientists in different parts of the world made a parallel discovery and identified two distinct classes of lymphocytes, B and T cells, a profound finding that provided the organising principle of the adaptive immune system. The Australian immunologist, Jacques Miller, discovered the role of the *thymus* in the development of a specific lymphocyte population; this led to the identification of T lymphocytes as essential for fending off infection. Meanwhile, the US immunologist, Max Cooper's work led to the revelation that plasma cells are derived from B-lymphocytes, which develop in the *bursa fabricii* in birds and in the bone marrow of mammals. B cells naturally produce monoclonal antibodies. Collectively, these discoveries accelerated the process of translational medicine and launched the course of modern immunology; now that the major cells of the immune response had been identified, immunologists increasingly focused on their biological functions.

Godal's scientific interests drew him to study the immunology of intracellular bacteria and cell-mediated immunity; later in Jon Lamvik's laboratory, at the Gades Institute in Bergen, he learned how to cultivate lymphocytes. Bergen has been called 'the cradle of modern leprosy', and a nineteenth-century native of the city, the physician Daniel Cornelius Danielssen was known as 'the father of leprology'.[14] It was Danielssen's son-in-law, Gerhard Henrik Armauer Hansen, who discovered the leprosy bacillus, *Mycobacterium laprae*, in 1873.[15] Hansen's name is immortalised in the medical taxonomy, as leprosy is also known as Hansen's disease (HD). Leprosy in Norway, as in most of Europe, dates back to the early medieval period, but it was in the nineteenth century that Norway led the world in the epidemiological, pathological and clinical understanding of the disease. This marked the beginning of the biologic knowledge of leprosy; clearly, Godal was following in a celebrated scientific tradition, and the focus of his laboratory work was becoming apparent – to unravel the mysteries of immunisation through the study of leprosy and other human diseases.

In 1969, Godal left Norway, to take up a postdoctoral position at the UK Medical Research Council's National Institute of Medical Research (NIMR), London, with R. J. W. 'Dick' Rees, a world expert on leprosy and Head of the Medical Research Council Laboratory for Leprosy Research. Working with Dick Rees introduced Godal to the pragmatic difficulties of how science and society can develop new treatments for diseases that are commercially unattractive to pharmaceutical companies, and deliver existing therapies to the very poorest and most deprived peoples of the world. Within the dynamic scientific environment of the NIMR, he also met the Australian parasitologist, Bridget Ogilvie, who would later become the Director of the Wellcome Trust, Europe's richest medical charity; and in 1999, the first Chair of Medicines for Malaria Venture, an early exemplar of innovative Public–Private Partnerships set up to develop new therapies for neglected infectious diseases.

For some people, the work they do and the life they lead are in perfect alignment. The biologist and socialist, Philip D'Arcy Hart, achieved this dazzling symmetry, and was one of the most inspiring figures that Godal met at the NIMR in Mill Hill. In 1965, at the age of 65, after a lifetime of pioneering work conducting epidemiological research and clinical trials, Hart turned entirely to laboratory studies on *Mycobacterium*, a genus known to cause diseases including tuberculosis and leprosy. Hart was a leading authority on tuberculosis, and after World War II, together with a young TB researcher, Marc Daniels, and the statistician Bradford Hill, was responsible for conducting an investigation into the therapeutic efficacy of streptomycin as a treatment for TB. This became one of the most celebrated randomised clinical trials in medical history.[16] Later assessments of remedies or combinations of drugs followed the same methodology as the streptomycin trial, and the MRC's Tuberculosis Research Unit, under Hart's direction, focused on developing the statistical design and analysis of therapeutic trials.[17] Hart was a modern-thinking, idealist physician, who campaigned in the

1930s for the UK National Health Service, which was eventually established in 1948, and he was part of a group of who were determined to make what the Marxist historian Henry Sigerist[18] described as a 'people's war for health'.[19] Godal learned much from Philip D'Arcy Hart about the politics and the science of evidence-based medicine, and importantly, this commitment to the health of others would be a lifelong pursuit. Philip D'Arcy Hart retained the status of an Attached Worker at the NIMR, until his death at the age of 106, on 30 July 2006.

During the final months of Godal's specialist training at the NIMR, he worked with Avrion 'Av' Mitchison's immunology group where he studied the recent discoveries in the new immunology, particularly the unearthing of T- and B-lymphocytes. Many discovery scientists thought Mill Hill to be the centre of the immunological universe, and once Godal understood the biological function of T cells, he knew it would be theoretically possible to make vaccines against neglected tropical diseases. In the laboratories at Mill Hill, he saw how critically important research and development (R&D) into health was if the causes of the major diseases in poor countries were to be addressed. Having gained some knowledge of the science of immunology, he was determined to apply it in Ethiopia and, in addition to this scientific approach, he was equally determined to implement programmes designed to reduce the fear and stigma associated with leprosy. In 1970, this holistic attitude to what is widely recognised as one of the most dreaded of all human diseases would serve him well when he left Norway with his wife Kari, and their children, to begin his innovatory work in global health.

The Armauer Hansen Research Institute (AHRI) was founded in 1969 as an independent international institute for biomedical research, with much of the funding coming through a joint initiative of the Norwegian and Swedish 'Save the Children' organisations allied to the Ethiopian Ministry of Health.[20] Located in Addis Ababa close to the All Africa Leprosy Rehabilitation and Training Centre (ALERT), with a hospital serving some ten million inhabitants, the concept of AHRI was to develop an integrated combination of leprosy patient care, field control, research, training and rehabilitation.[21] Today, the AHRI is a bustling biomedical enterprise with over 350 researchers, and as a scientific centre of excellence within Africa, it forms an important axis upon which global health partnerships turn. However, when Godal arrived in the summer of 1970, the entire AHRI workforce was in single figures; fortunately, they did have a modern and well-equipped laboratory in which to work, that had been established by his predecessor, Morten Harboe. For his part, Godal was conscious that there was much to play for, and that the stakes were high – not only was he forging a new career in tropical medicine, the Armauer Hansen Research Institute constituted a great national experiment, as it marked the first time that Norway was directly involved in medical research in Africa. Godal's closest collaborator during the three years he was in Ethiopia became Bjørn Myrvang an MD PHD student from Norway. Myrvang had arrived in Ethiopia in 1969 with Professor Harboe and his doctoral thesis is entitled *Immune Responses to Mycobacterium Leprae in Man*. 'I had never seen a leprosy patient until I arrived in Addis', recalled Bjørn Myrvang, 'it was a very creative time in my life. Tore and I worked closely together, he supervised my thesis, and was co-author on all of my papers, and I think we wrote about 10 papers together.[22] It all started there in Addis – we were pioneers!'[23]

Addis Ababa was a resonant counterpoint to Godal's life in rural Norway, and there is no doubt that the three years he spent working and travelling in Ethiopia gave him an insight into the difficulties that researchers in the field had to overcome on a daily basis. Heat, humidity, poor roads, fragile health systems, working under extremely difficult conditions, all of these elements shaped his thinking and the subsequent design of how he thought cost-effective health programmes could realistically evolve in low- and middle-income countries. Early in his career, Godal came to understand that global health and effective research in tropical diseases had to make sense to the health worker, toiling in some remote village in a very poor country. Godal wasn't interested in highfalutin speeches about 'humanity', what interested him was how the World Health Organisation, UNICEF, and the international community could translate ideals and ideas into constructive actions, therapeutics and drugs on the ground to help people in tangible ways. In this respect, the experiences of three years that he spent in Ethiopia lasted a lifetime.

Throughout his life, Tore Godal has been strongly addicted to work; it was a compulsion he shared with Armauer Hansen. Johanne Margrethe Tideman, Hansen's second wife, even said that her husband 'was more interested in his research than his home',[24] and in 1970 when Godal arrived in the laboratory, 'he was very hard working and full of ideas'.[25] The origins of his research usually derived from clinical observations and, together with others, he investigated how immune system reactions exacerbate nerve damage in leprosy patients.[26] He also identified key immune mechanisms involved in the clinical and sub-clinical manifestations of leprosy.[27] These studies established his reputation as a brilliant investigator, and a steady stream of researchers sought opportunities to work with him at the AHRI. Again, working with his colleague, Bjorn Myvang, Godal identified the immunological response (T-cell responses to M-leprae) in patients with leprosy was more important than the bacterial infection. These insightful observations drew international attention, and in the autumn of 1972, Godal was invited to a World Health Organisation Expert Committee meeting in Geneva on the subject of 'Cell-mediated immunity and resistance to infection'. The Australian immunologist, George B. Mackaness, an expert in anti-infection immunology and TB, chaired the meeting. The gathering coincided with the great surge into research in molecular and cell biology, and it also brought together a group of scientists that, through a combination of basic and applied research, were to fundamentally alter the trajectory of tropical disease medicine. Another member of the new generation of researchers attending the conference was Barry Bloom, an immunologist at Albert Einstein College of Medicine, New York City. After the meeting ended, over drinks at an evening reception, Godal had a long talk with Bloom about his research in Ethiopia and the lessons that the science of immunology could learn from leprosy.[28] This proved a fateful encounter for both researchers and began a lasting scientific collaboration and friendship. Although not medically qualified, Bloom wanted to use science to improve human health by understanding the causes and finding novel treatments for infectious diseases. As Bloom's laboratory studies of cellular immune reactions became increasingly accepted as a legitimate immunological endeavour, he was invited to the WHO meeting to help evaluate whether these emerging laboratory-based, in vitro techniques might have some practical relevance to understanding immunity to tropical diseases.

> I had discovered cytokines, and Howard Goodman, head of immunology at WHO, thought it was the cure for leprosy, and he organised a meeting in Geneva of three scientists who knew nothing about leprosy, and three or four leprologists who knew nothing about science – and Tore, who was able to link the two. Tore introduced me to the health problems of what was then termed the *Third World* and the problem of leprosy from which I have never quite recovered.[29]

The discussion changed the direction of Bloom's research, and the immunology of mycobacteria became a leading focus of his research throughout the rest of his career.

The Birth of TDR

One of the elements responsible for the renaissance of interest in the ancient disease of leprosy in the 1960s and 1970s was the extraordinary possibilities it offered for gaining insight into the regulation of the immune system. Intriguingly, leprosy is not a single clinical entity, but rather a spectral disease that presents a diversity of clinical manifestations. At one end of the spectrum, with tuberculoid leprosy, patients develop high levels of specific cell-mediated immunity that ultimately kills and clears the bacteria in the tissue, although often accompanied by damage to the nerves. At the other spectrum range is lepromatous leprosy, where patients exhibit a selective unresponsiveness to antigens of the leprosy bacteria, the organisms multiply in the skin, and it becomes a progressive disease.[30] In his position as director of the AHRI, Godal was in the vanguard of the scientific understanding of both the pathogenesis of the disease and, just as importantly, to its treatment. Crucially, his experiences in Ethiopia cemented a profound understanding of what life was really like for people living in abject poverty, and how the lives of the poor were perpetually blighted by diseases that were effectively caused *by* poverty and responsible *for* the causes of poverty. This realisation inspired in him a determination to try to integrate the social and biomedical sciences and an appreciation of the critical need for an interdisciplinary approach to help solve health problems.[31] Godal's combination of fitting in and standing out caught the attention of the host of the meeting in Geneva, the US immunologist Howard C. Goodman. At the time, there was no international research framework for infectious disease control in the developing world; but in 1970, with the establishment of the WHO Immunology and Leprosy research programme, a new era was evident within the corridors of power in Geneva. This change came, in part, as a response to the growing belief that the new biomedical sciences of immunology, biology, genetics and molecular medicine could transform human health; and partly, because of a call from The World Health Assembly for the Director-General of the WHO to 'intensify WHO activities in tropical disease research'.[32] In the politics of global health, as in life, timing is a determining factor; in 1973, the visionary health idealist, Halfdan Mahler was elected Director-General of WHO. Mahler, who had spent a decade in India developing the country's national tuberculosis programme, shared with Godal and Goodman a belief that poverty caused illness and that much disease was caused by social, economic and other environmental factors.[33] At the epicentre of this expanding philosophy of world health was Howard Goodman and his 'small band of immunologists'[34] who wanted to provide new strategies for dealing with the fundamental public health problems of developing countries. Godal's dedication to science and his promotion of research training at the AHRI impressed Goodman to such a degree that he offered Tore a one-year consultancy with the WHO's Immunology Unit in Geneva. This was to be a propitious time in Godal's career, and it helped to usher in a new and exciting era in tropical disease medicine. Before taking up his post, however, he first had to return to Addis Ababa to complete his three-year tenure as director of the Armauer Hansen Research Institute.

The lived experience of Ethiopia, in addition to changing Godal's world view, marked an inflection point in the arc of his career, with a commitment to use science to cure the devastating diseases of poverty;[35] but the country also had a profound influence on the lives of his children and his wife, Kari. The oldest children joined the 'Jack and Jill Nursery' where they integrated happily into their new life. Indeed, it was Kari, a language student at the time, who was to make a lasting contribution to the ethos of 'rehabilitation', one of the foundational cornerstones of the institute. Kari, recalls Bjørn Myrvang

was very important in that connection. She worked with patients who had handicaps, and ran weaving, knitting, embroidery and sewing classes. The workshop still exists I think. . . . It was not part of the institute, it was part of ALERT – Kari did very important work during her stay in Addis.[36]

When Barry Bloom visited the AHRI to work with Godal in the lab, he witnessed Kari's skilled and sensitive teaching.

> I saw her with leprosy patients, and I remember women who had no fingers skilfully embroidering. I adored Kari, she was very interested in Nordic mythology, she was gentle and caring and I saw her working miracles with people in her workshop.[37]

This work vividly displayed the delicate skills of patients, and contributed to an African-based experiment that sought to remove the mystery, legend and attribution of moral taint that had degraded the disease throughout much of human history.[38] One of the common features in the literature of leprosy is the stigmatisation of the disease, and the All-African training centre for leprosy rehabilitation, known as ALERT, opened in Addis Ababa in 1966, and weathered social, political, funding and famine crisis before growing as 'a living organism' into the twenty-first century.[39]

According to one of his closest colleagues, when Godal left the Hansen Institute in 1973, Ethiopia had become, 'very close to his heart',[40] and during the preceding three years, scientifically he had done much to advance the biological understanding of the disease.[41] At the age of 34, Godal had found his calling, and the World Health Organisation had now given him the opportunity to do something meaningful for patients with the scientific knowledge that he had accumulated. This commitment by scientists to improve human development in developing countries by investigating, eliminating and eradicating some of nature's most debilitating infectious diseases would later be described poetically by Godal as, 'the *conscience* of science'.[42]

When Godal arrived in Geneva, Howard Goodman was already developing an ambitious programme to focus biomedical research on the diseases of the developing countries and provide new strategies for dealing with public health problems. In 1974, the World Health Assembly endorsed Halfdan Mahler's proposal for intensifying research on tropical diseases, and approved plans for a Special Programme for Research and Training in Tropical Diseases. Strenuous efforts followed to reassure African countries this was not another post-colonial construct; that the programme should strengthen the research capability of developing countries, and crucially, Mahler allowed recruitment of staff on 'merit', which enabled the programme to resist the political and bureaucratic pressures to select staff on other criteria.[43] During the early evolution of what became the UNDP/World Bank/WHO Special Programme for Research and Training in Tropical Diseases – or TDR for short – disagreements over its design, strategy approach, and choice of diseases threatened its survival.[44] The complications surrounding TDR's operational strategy eased when the Swedish Noble laureate and influential global health ambassador Sune Bergstrom suggested a change in operational policy from an institution-based to a network approach.[45] Having rejected the international research institute model, as high-risk and capital-intensive, Bergstrom proposed a novel design involving international networks of collaborating centres. The component elements of the network acting jointly would provide the critical mass for achieving the specific goals of the programme. Two years earlier, in 1972, the network approach had been successfully established by Bergstrom and the Canadian tropical disease physician, Richard Wilson when they collaborated on the WHO Human Reproduction Programme. To establish the network approach, Bergstrom looked around for an idea in tropical disease medicine that could act as a template for TDR and synthesise the evolving disciplines of immunology and molecular biology. At the time, Godal was working on 'a plan to develop a leprosy vaccine through a network approach', a concept that arose out his research on the ability of T cells to annihilate virus-infected cells and support the production of antibodies.[46] On one of his many visits to Geneva, Bergstrom visited Godal and when he saw the detailed plans taking shape, he said, 'We need to start a pilot project, and I suggest we start with the immunology of leprosy'.[47] Bergstrom's scientific expertise was not his only talent; in addition, he had great political acumen and practised in the art of the persuasive late evening phone call to ensure his ideas were successful.

IMMLEP

Godal's industriousness had developed a strategy to advance the immunology of leprosy with the aim of developing a vaccine against the disease. The favoured candidate was a killed leprosy bacilli mixed with BCG (the TB vaccine) as an adjuvant to make it work more effectively. It rapidly became clear to Godal that to find the most fruitful areas for immunologic exploration would require a network of institutions in both the developed north and the geographical south. This included supporting the research of Eleanor Storrs in Louisiana, US, who discovered that the bacillus grew abundantly when injected into nine-banded armadillos and raised the possibility of developing an armadillo-derived vaccine.[48] He identified a need to fund researchers working on leprosy in experimental animals such as Charles Shepard at CDC in Atlanta, US, and his colleague Dick Rees from Mill Hill, London. Moreover, he also selected the work of one of the world's great pioneers in leprosy vaccine strategy, Dr Jacinto Convit, in Caracas, Venezuela. Godal's network went on to include the AHRI and basic immunology in Morten Harboe's laboratory in Oslo and Barry Bloom's laboratory in New York City. Bloom was instrumental in identifying and attracting the best scientists into the field including the molecular biologists Richard Young and Ron Davis at Stanford, who joined to make recombinant genomic libraries and eventually sequenced the leprosy bacilli.[49] A decisive moment in the nascent history of TDR occurred when Norway donated US$57,000 to establish a pilot programme, named 'The Immunology of Leprosy Scientific Working Group' (IMMLEP) as it represented the first donation to TDR. The dynamic within TDR came from the 'conscience' of scientists, and IMMLEP illustrated the degree to which world-leading researchers were willing to dedicate their careers to finding treatments for the diseases affecting the poorest countries in the world.

In July 1974, at the International Congress of Immunology in Brighton (UK), the leading Australian immunologist, Gus Nossal gave a moving speech appealing to his colleagues to take on the challenges of tropical diseases and apply the recent advances in basic immunology to eliminate the causes of much avoidable human suffering. Nossal was deeply involved in the political aspects of medical health and, in 1976, he spent one year in Geneva planning the scientific programme with Howard Goodman and later with the Nigerian physician, Adetokunbo Lucas, who succeeded Goodman as director of TDR in 1976. Nossal's participation helped to put TDR on a strong scientific footing, and when the programme was launched in 1976, the six diseases selected for investigation were malaria, schistosomiasis, filariasis, trypanosomiasis, leishmaniosis and leprosy. In recognition of Godal's scientific leadership of IMMLEP, leprosy was the only bacterial disease chosen; all of the others were parasitic infections. The diseases were selected based on their public health impact, and some of the choices were contentious. Why, for example, was leishmaniosis included, while tuberculosis with its high levels of mortality excluded? Rather than Machiavellian intrigue or the power of medico-political lobbying, the explanation, according to Adetokunbo O. Lucas, 'probably had more to do with the fascination of immunologists with the biology of the parasite than with clear conviction that it merited action on the basis of the morbidity and mortality attributed to these infections'.[50] However, according to Chris Murray, a founder of the Global Burden of Disease (GBD),[51] other determinants influenced the neglected status of tuberculosis.

> The lore was that Mahler viewed TB as hopeless because of his experiences in India and there wasn't much to be done. Therefore, the disease was very much downplayed, and people did not think of TB as a 'tropical disease' it is a universal disease. . . . The perception was that it was a disease of 'older men' and so it did not affect the mood of 'tropical diseases affecting younger people' . . . That was a good part of the reason for it not being one of the diseases selected by TDR. I also think that Mahler thought it would be hard to raise money for TB.[52]

Nonetheless, this was a providential time for the practice of the subspecialty, and WHO was not the only institution beginning to think more about the application of first-class, high-powered science to tropical diseases. In the United States, private philanthropy led the way and the Edna McConnell Clark Foundation, under its director, Joseph A. Cook, was to play a leading role in research into schistosomiasis and trachoma. Of even great significance was the work of Kenneth. S. Warren, Director of Health Sciences at the Rockefeller Foundation, who in 1978

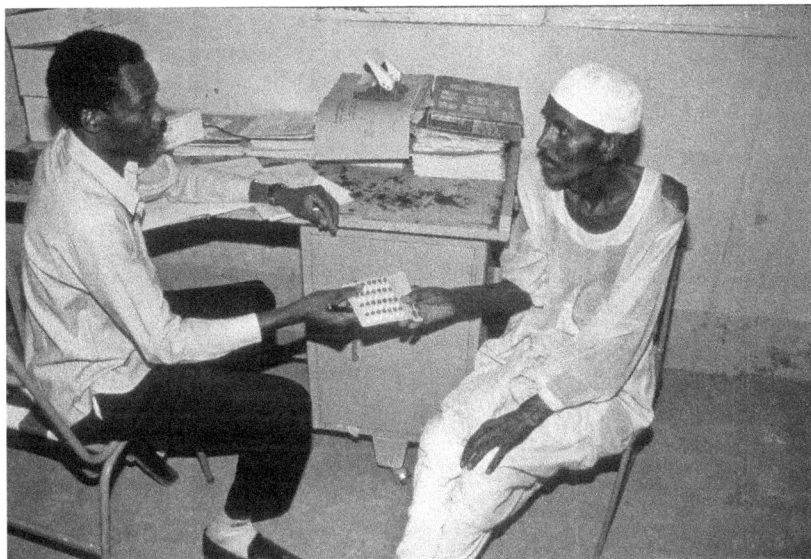

Figure 1.1 A doctor treating a man with leprosy in Sudan in 1997. It is worth remembering that it can take many years, sometimes many decades, between the discovery of an infectious agent and the development of a vaccine capable of controlling a disease. The polio vaccine took almost 50 years to develop, while a malaria vaccine needed almost 150 years to reach patients. There is still no effective leprosy vaccine.

Source: Courtesy of Andy Crump.

launched a network of research laboratories devoted to the study of tropical diseases. Warren was a powerful and polarising figure and his programme '*The Great Neglected Diseases of Mankind*' was designed to attract scientists working in 'highly sophisticated laboratories'[53] in immunology, genetics and molecular medicine to apply their knowledge to infectious diseases of the poor.[54] Warren, a larger than life character, from what was essentially a financially modest power-base, revolutionised tropical disease research.[55] His approach was individualistic, impulsive, dogmatic and original. In fact, temperamentally Warren represented a vivid contrast to Godal's measured, judicious and diplomatic approach; and while their modus operandi differed greatly, collectively their work transformed the tropical disease movement and gave it scientific credibility. On the global level, both of these influential tropical disease physicians agreed that the support for health in the developing world was grossly inadequate, but this policy equipoise did not prevent Warren from criticising TDR's disease portfolio that 'developed a programme of research on the diseases of the tropics which omitted diarrhoeal and respiratory infections'.[56] Of course, countries, physicians, politicians and international agencies can have emotional and historical attachments to specific diseases, in Godal's case it was to leprosy; and for Warren, it was to the parasitic disease schistosomiasis. Moreover, there was much common ground, and both the Rockefeller Foundation and TDR selected malaria in their disease portfolios; but for the British epidemiologist, Richard Peto, there were also emotional, philosophical and economic forces at play in the difficult art and science of setting health priorities.

> I think Ken rubbed Tore up the wrong way in all sorts of ways, but on the other hand he had some respect for him as well. I do not know what Tore's opinion of Ken is. . . . But, I do think that the work Ken co-authored, '*Good Health at Low Cost*',[57] which asked the question 'how many lives will be saved for money spent' was a useful perspective, and was later taken forward by Dean Jamison, and the World Bank, and drew attention to the cost-effectiveness of vaccines, and similar low-cost interventions against pneumonia and diarrhoeal diseases.[58]

Unquestionably, Godal was one of the first scientific administrators to realise that WHO was ineffective in doing research, and IMMLEP was a successful forerunner of TDR; having an independent governance from WHO with its own

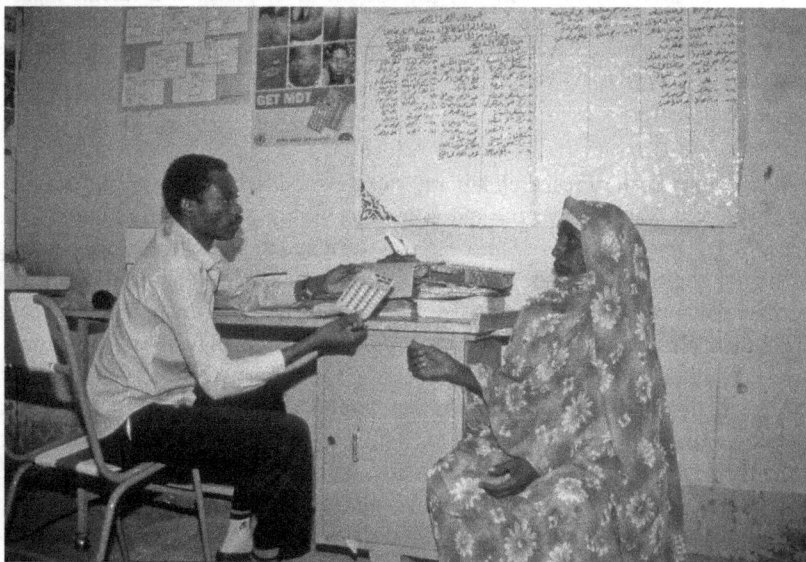

Figure 1.2 A doctor giving multi-drug treatment (MDT) packs to a female patient in what is now South Sudan. The MDT packs were provided free by the pharmaceutical corporation Novartis and distributed under the WHO guidance.

Source: Courtesy of Andy Crump.

advisory committee structure, and crucially, independent funding while being insulated from WHO's political and bureaucratic manipulation.[59] From the beginning, TDR was an early adopter of 'translational research' and 'product development' in the treatment of disease. In the case of leprosy, the group tasked with developing drugs for treating the disease was THELEP – an acronym of (drug) therapy for leprosy.[60] THELEP's existence was as a direct response to a major problem that began to appear in the 1970s; this was the emergence of drug-resistant strains of leprosy to the antibiotic dapsone, which had been the drug of choice for two decades. In order to understand the extent of antimicrobial resistance, THELEP initiated studies in different parts of the world; these showed that there was indeed widespread resistance to dapsone's use as a monotherapy for leprosy. In response, THELEP developed a strategy to use a combination of drugs, known as multi-drug therapy (MDT) to reduce the risk that leprosy bacteria would develop resistance. Luis M. Bechelli, the Brazilian head of the leprosy unit at WHO, stubbornly resisted all of TDR's calls for moving from a monotherapy to multiple drug therapy. However, in 1981, a new head of leprosy at WHO, a French physician, Hubert Sansarricq, understood the clarity of the statistical evidence from the clinical trials, and recommended MDT as a safe, effective and easily administered treatment, even before the trials were completed.[61] TDR rapidly brought about a transformation in the epidemiology of leprosy. In the 1970s, ten to 12 million people suffered from the disease, and there was little hope of a cure. By the 1990s, the success of MDT had led to a fourfold reduction in the disease. For the first time in human history, it was possible to prevent and cure leprosy.

A Norwegian Interregnum

For the period of 12 years between 1974 and 1986, Godal was Director of Immunology at Oslo's Radium Hospital. While working at this tertiary hospital his team observed the potential of immunotherapy for cancer treatment, 'even though it took a further three decades before it became a clinical reality', he told *The Lancet* in 2019.[62] These were prodigious years for Godal. As a lead cancer immunological investigator, he helped to develop new diagnostic tools and produce monoclonal antibodies for use in the classification, prognosis and treatment of leukaemia and lymph node cancer.[63] Meanwhile, he retained his leadership of IMMLEP until 1981 and continued working in tropical medicine, as a delegate of Norway on the powerful Joint Coordinating Board (JCB) of TDR, and specifically on the immunopathology and epidemiology of mycobacteria.[64] To become a leading researcher in even one area of biomedical science is an extraordinary achievement, but to achieve that distinction simultaneously in the fields of non-infectious and infectious disease research is rare. Initially educated in a one-room schoolhouse by one teacher, Godal only went to school on alternate days during the years of World War II. When Bill Foege, the epidemiologist who devised the global strategy that led to the eradication of small pox, learned of this, he would to tease his friend about 'how much could he learn if he only when to school half time?'[65] The answer was that Godal's uncushioned childhood had taught him the transformative power of determined action, and the convergence of his ethical upbringing, and medical training, fostered in him an attitude of casual intensity, in which a relaxed and approachable personal style disguised an unstinting drive. This intellectual energy allowed Godal to stay at the forefront of tropical disease medical thinking[66] and retain contact with a network of scientific collaborators across disciplines and continents even while living and working in Norway.

Global Leadership

TDR had started with a major focus on Africa, the continent where the disease burden was greatest, and the research and development capability lowest. Following Godal's three years in Ethiopia, Africa had become, according to Helga Fogstad, a global health colleague, 'very close to his heart';[67] and his vision for organising research and development for infectious diseases was that programme activities must provide 'a *complete pipeline* from strategic research to applied field research'.[68] This programmatic philosophy, coupled with his diplomatic stewardship of IMMLEP, gave him credibility with the WHO hierarchy, and especially with the Director-General Halfdan Mahler, who viewed Godal as a trusted, politically savvy global health administrator, and one capable of making people work together. In 1986, Adetokunbo Lucas's widely acclaimed ten-year leadership of TDR[69] ended, and Godal succeeded him as director of TDR. Godal's management of scientific programmes and his ability to learn from the past and anticipate the future made him a natural successor to Adetokunbo O. Lucas. Of course, his accession to the directorship of TDR meant much more than merely ascending a summit of global health governance. His friend and ally, Helga Fogstad believes that when Godal went to Ethiopia in 1970, it was 'because he wanted to save the world in Africa',[70] but no one should mistake him for a romantic idealist, his idealism took a very different form. He wanted to shape TDR into a global force to combat diseases of poverty through the rational application of science, innovation and cost-effective programmes.[71] In addition to funding research on the problems that affect poor countries, Godal wanted TDR to build capacity in those countries for conducting research themselves and refute the idea that health research was something rich countries did and then exported knowledge, in a colonial manner, to the poor regions of the world. 'The goal must be', Godal wrote 'for risk-benefit decisions to be made as close as possible to the populations at risk – and ideally by that population'.[72]

When Godal arrived in the TDR building in Geneva, he set about building the institution 'from the bottom up'.[73] The dynamic within TDR would come from young scientists, and his philosophy was to find the most able people, support them to the best of his ability and trust in their judgement. He also wanted TDR to be a lean organisation, because at the institutional level he understood the reality of the Indian proverb, 'nothing grows under a Banyan tree'. The way ahead would be through the rationale of increased innovation and reduced bureaucracy. To achieve this aim, Godal deployed the astute operational skills of Sue Tyrrell and her knowledge and experience of the Darwinian world of WHO politics. In his memoir, Adetokunbo O. Lucas wrote, 'Ms Susan Block, now Block-Tyrrell, became a dynamic manager in TDR. Her recruitment turned out to be one of the most important decisions that I make as director of TDR',[74] as the public relations touchstone of the programme Block-Tyrrell offers a unique insight into the contrasting personal and managerial styles of the two directors.

> I got on extremely well with both of them – but there was a cultural change, and management styles were completely different. Going from a very vibrant, joking but serious and professional Nigerian to a typical Viking Norwegian . . . Tore was a good listener. He would listen, and then he would come in with his views. He had the amazing knack to being able to recognise what was needed in global public health, and try to figure out how he and TDR could fill that gap and get things done. Even after he left TDR, this remained a feature of his work in global health. He was always one-step ahead.[75]

Arguably, one of TDR's foremost achievements in advancing public health and training a critical mass of African researchers transcended the contiguous directorships of Lucas and Godal. This was the history shaping collaboration between TDR and the US pharmaceutical company Merck to build a programme, founded on donating a drug free of charge, to eliminate onchocerciasis (also known as river blindness), in Africa and other geographies. The initial negotiations led ably by Dr Lucas then passed to Godal in 1986. These discussions ultimately led to the first programme that sought to unite pharmaceutical companies, donors and endemic countries in a commitment to control eliminate or eradicate a neglected tropical disease; and was the template for 2012 London Declaration that expanded this philanthropic commitment to ten diseases affecting over one billion people. (The more detailed river blindness story is discussed in Chapter 2.)

From the outset, Godal's objective was 'to get things done'.[76] He immediately moved TDR away from the 'investigator-driven disease focus', towards 'product development' and 'applied field research'. The Merck negotiations had galvanised his belief in the crucial need for equitable and comprehensive collaborations between the private and public sectors, even if it led to some internal political turbulence and turf wars within the corridors of WHO. One invaluable element that allowed him, in the main, to sidestep the Machiavellian intrigue of WHO politics was the supportive relationship that he enjoyed with Halfdan Mahler. Culturally and philosophically, they had much in common; both their fathers had been Lutheran pastors (Adetokunbo Lucas's father was also a clergyman); they had a professional interest in bacterial diseases; and as Scandinavians, their beliefs, mores and world view were formed by a shared historical experience.

In comparison to the directors of the control programmes funded by the regular WHO budget, Godal was financially autonomous, having access to an annual revenue stream of approximately $100,000 million in today's value. This allowed him to incubate many programmes inside TDR that drew people's attention to the diffuse areas of the economic and social research of tropical diseases, gender issues and the psychological aspects of sequelae, while his scientific background ensured that TDR pursued the development of vaccines for leishmaniasis, malaria and leprosy.[77] In the early 1970s, there was great excitement in the leprosy world when Eleanor Storrs, who had a lifelong interest in armadillos, discovered that the bacillus grew abundantly when injected into nine-banded armadillos, whose body temperature is a few degrees lower than that of humans. This raised the possibility of developing a leprosy vaccine based on leprosy bacilli grown in armadillos, from which bacilli could be harvested, and then killed, and purified. The organisation of large-scale trials of an armadillo-derived vaccine became a major activity of TDR and IMMLEP. In the late 1980s and early 1990s, three large clinical trials took place in Venezuela, Malawi and South India in which killed leprosy bacilli were mixed with BCG. These trials were a massive undertaking, involving tens of thousands of participants; unfortunately, the results were disappointing with no evidence of protection in Venezuela and Malawi, but what they did show was TDR's ability to coordinate large-scale field trials in developing countries. This expertise was successfully built upon with lasting effect, when multidisciplinary teams simultaneously tested the impact and effectiveness of insecticide-impregnated bednets (ITNs) against malaria in several sub-Saharan countries. TDR funded these randomised controlled trials, and ITNs have formed the cornerstone of malaria control for the past 30 years (the full story of malaria can be read in Chapter 3). One of the team working across these studies was the Australian economist, David Evans, who joined TDR in 1990.

> Whether it was a malaria vaccine, or the leprosy vaccine, or insecticide bednets, Tore always said the same thing, 'we have to know if it works'. My research spanned all of the diseases: trying to understand why people were not availing themselves of the technologies that were available, examining what were the barriers to access, seeing if people were willing to use bednets, and determining what type of house improvements could make them more resistant to the sand-fly vector of leishmaniasis. Tore liked my work, and he was a big supporter of integrating social and biomedical sciences.[78]

By its very nature, biomedical research advances incrementally, but in the case of malaria vaccines, the discovery of the circumsporozoite protein (CSP) in the 1980s set in motion a worldwide race to make a malaria vaccine. As the world's most lethal disease and the biggest killer of children in Africa, Godal was eager to promote malaria vaccine research at a time when comparatively few researchers were working on the infection. In 1987, it appeared that a vaccine developed by the Columbian physician Manuel Patarroyo looked promising and his claims to have developed and tested a vaccine in South America initiated a major controversy within the malaria community in the United Kingdom, the United States and other developed countries – between those who would not accept that a Columbian working in Columbia could have developed the world's first malaria vaccine, and others, like Godal and Brian Greenwood, who considered that it should be given a chance, and evaluated in Africa. Alas, when the vaccine was tested in a randomised controlled trial in Africa, the results were disappointing. At the time, Patarroyo was seen by some researchers as a controversial figure,[79] a bit of a showman and over-ambitious, but this is not unique in the malaria world and Brian Greenwood believes that Patarroyo deserves recognition for what he tried to do, as his was not the first malaria vaccine to have failed.[80] For his part, Godal knew that discovery science was a fusion of black holes and revelations, and it is not possible to know in advance where innovation is going to come from. He was unafraid of failure; his responsibility as a leader of tropical disease research was to 'know if it works'.

New Global Partnerships

TDR's determination to harness research and development to reduce the global burden of disease led to innovative associations often referred to as global public–private partnerships (PPPs). The goal of these partnerships was to grow effective interactions with big pharmaceutical companies that would fast-track product development in the form of diagnostics and cost-effective drugs. Because resistance had developed to chloroquine and Sulphadoxine/pyramethamine, the cheap and previously effective antimalarial drugs, Godal was scanning the horizon looking for ways to develop new and much-needed therapies for the world's most deadly infectious disease. A decisive moment in his attempts to resuscitate the pharmaceutical industry's commitment to antimalarial drugs came when he recruited Win Gutteridge from Burrows Wellcome Research Laboratories to become TDR's chief of product research and development. Gutteridge, a successful translational researcher who had developed Malarone for the treatment of malaria, found working within the WHO framework too constraining[81] and that the early promise of WHO/TDR to develop new therapies was not paying off. Consequently, Gutteridge became a driving force behind Medicines for Malaria Venture (MMV) a pioneering global (PPP). These types of partnerships have expanded exponentially since the 1990s, bringing together international agencies, the private and public sectors, non-governmental organisations (NGOs), and civil society, to provide a more practical approach to solving global problems.[82] MMV also reunited Godal with Bridget Ogilvie, a colleague from the

National Institute of Medical Research, who became the first chair of MMV in 1999 and who shared his vision to 'discover, develop and deliver new antimalarial drugs'.[83] MMV's early success was in bringing together academia, pharma and those with experience in the field in a very positive way. It grew from a small group of dedicated individuals with ambition, to become, in the opinion of the malariologist, Brian Greenwood, 'one of the most successful PPPs and a driving force in malaria drug development'.[84] Arguably, the development of new antimalarial drugs has been disappointing given the substantial investment in MMV, but the process of developing new antimalarials has been exacting, and MMV has recruited high-quality people directly from the pharmaceutical industry with experience in discovery science. Today, MMV has over 20 antimalarial drugs in the pipeline with several promising candidates and an annual income of over US$60 million.[85] However, it cannot go unnoticed that the three fundamental cornerstones of malaria control – long-lasting insecticide-treated nets, rapid diagnostic tests and artemisinin-based combination therapies – were all developed in the 1980s and 1990s. Indeed, many of the Product Development Partnerships (PDPs) that target economically deprived markets have in the main, failed to deliver new groundbreaking treatments. After more than two decades, it is now surely time for a sober assessment of the cost-effectiveness of investing in MMV and other similar organisations.

The camaraderie that flowed between Godal and Bridget Ogilvie, together with their collective determination to develop new treatments for the diseases of the very poorest and most deprived communities, helped to usher in a new era in global health. The advent of the Bill and Melinda Gates Foundation, the global health networks of The Wellcome Trust in Asia and Africa, and the emergence of pharmaco-philanthropic ventures in NTDs were a response to the rapidly changing, globalised world at the end of the twentieth century. The challenge for international public health directors like Godal was to understand, listen and connect with this world of private donors and the political sector, so as to bring about a revolution in public health.

As a communicator, Godal's style is straight talking, clear and very direct. On occasion, this direct approach led to feathers being ruffled, and WHO toes being stepped on, and he took pride in his reputation of being a steamroller, because when he wanted something done, his tactic was to just keep relentlessly moving forward.[86] Godal liked to move things quickly; 'speed is of the essence' was his mantra at TDR. One of his acknowledged skills was the ability to keep the donors happy, 'and keep them on side'.[87] He did this by being sincere and honest. He was also tireless in staying in contact with the main movers and shakers in global health, a talent that allowed him to see which way the winds were blowing and to build durable alliances with USAID, the Gates Foundation, DFID and other important donors. As a public speaker, Tore Godal is not one of the accomplished orators of global health – there are many of those – in contrast, he comes across as being serious and earnest. For example, often he might begin a lecture with a stanza from some impenetrable Norwegian poem, or with a folksy Norwegian joke that invariably falls flat, but according to his friend Barry Bloom, 'people loved him for it, because it wasn't to impress you, it was to show his humility'.[88] David Evans supports this view and feels that his former boss's influence derives from an inner self-belief. 'I think Tore feels that he is helping the world and leaving it a better place. In international health, in WHO, I don't think there are many people I would say that about'.[89] To affect the world outside, Godal wanted to germinate policies within TDR to build a new global architecture for health.[90] However, he had the shrewd sense that internally institutions had collective personalities and psychologies, as if they were extended families. Consequently, he was protective of the younger scientists coming into TDR and sought to build on their enthusiasm and create a sense of excitement, purpose and righteous direction. It is also true to say that TDR was less overtly 'political' in the pejorative sense than WHO, and Godal had succeeded in moulding the institution into a cohesive scientific collective, greater than the sum of its parts. Sue Tyrrell was the public relations dynamo who ably assisted Godal throughout his 12 years as director and vividly describes the uniqueness of what it came to represent, 'TDR was such a special programme at the time, because it was the tall tree in the empty field'.[91] Godal had championed the policy that all research proposals seeking TDR funding would be evaluated by an independent expert committee; this had the dual advantage of avoiding the forces of nepotism that had increased under the new WHO Director-General, Hiroshi Nakajima, while advancing the ethos of impartiality in the Godal era.

After two years, it was already apparent what Godal had achieved. In 1990, Barry Bloom was the head of TDR's *Scientific and Technical Advisory Committee* (STAC) – his job was to attract first-rate scientist and get them to work on tropical diseases 'for very little money'. At one of the STAC meetings, the discussion turned to the only thing that counts when a research programme is being planned – where to put the money! What followed, according to Bloom, was unprecedented:

I've never seen anything like it. The committee was fantastic, when we had a vote; the basic scientists felt that there needed to be more money allocated to training and epidemiology, while the epidemiologists pressed for more investment in basic science, because they needed more tools to deal with the diseases. I almost wept. I have never seen people moved beyond their own self-interest as at that meeting. That was Tore's skill in creating something that I had never seen before.[92]

One of the elements that contributed to Godal's ability to shape a common bond with his colleagues was that he was widely considered as being without personal vanity, he made simple convincing arguments, and he built trust by being honest. The unconscious assimilation of the concept of building trust and the ideals of public service, equity and internationalism had begun in childhood and opened his mind to think about people living in distant geographies, beyond his valley home in Norway. In the intervening years, while he had lived much of his life in other countries, he remained quintessentially Norwegian and held true to those universal values learned in the village of Rauland. As the novelist F. Scott Fitzgerald constantly reminded himself, *action is character*, and for Godal, the memory of his father sheltering the resistance fighters before their attack on Nazi forces in Telemark reinforced in him an inescapable reality – the need to be prepared to do radical things if you want to change the world and get good things done.

The action taken by determined people in 1943 against the might of an occupying army became a type of guiding metaphor for Godal, and throughout his stewardship of TDR he knew that small players with integrity on their side could influence global health and enable people to live longer and healthier lives. Norway, a country with a population of just 5.7 million, continues to have a disproportionately big effect on health and is the seventh largest donor to the UN. Beginning in 1970, Norway took an active role in global health with its support for the AHRI, and the symbiosis between an utterly dedicated individual and a nation determined to 'fight poverty and work for a more just world',[93] led Chris Murray to this powerful observation: 'I think that part of the sustained commitment of Norway to health is due to Tore and not the other way round'.[94] What is certainly without question is that the drive to improve global health has been central to Norway's foreign policy programme. In this way, Norway has shown that a relatively small country with a foreign policy that is close to peoples' conscience can change global health thinking. As the director of TDR, Godal decided to hold an IMMLEP meeting in Rauland, his home village, in homage to the courageous actions of past generations and to celebrate Norway's involvement in tropical disease medicine. It proved poignant, because by a quirk of fate, the film showing in the small cinema in Rauland one evening was the 1965 Anthony Mann directed classic *The Heroes of Telemark*. The temptation was too great, and the STAC scientists led by Barry Bloom gathered to watch the film.

> Tore and I were cheering on Kirk Douglas to blow up the power plant. Of course, it was very emotional for Tore because of the actions of his father protecting those people. The film shows that there is a point beyond which you have to get it done. And Tore was very much in the mode of getting it done.[95]

Another influential researcher working in tropical disease medicine who had the convening power, money and vision to put together a network of highly motivated collaborators was the hyperthymic Kenneth S. Warren of the Rockefeller Foundation (RF). Both Godal and Warren needed finely tuned political skills if they were to survive and remain in control of their respective institutions, and at the time the RF's hierarchy were growing weary of Warren's methods and wanted to curb his autonomy. For almost a decade, TDR and the RF's *Great Neglected Diseases of Mankind Program* had been running in parallel, and while there had been ideological tensions between the systems, in 1986, they announced the establishment of a collaborative research programme to construct a global laboratory.[96] Warren's hope was that fusion of the RF's private-sector philanthropy with the WHO's humanitarianism would deflect the hesitancies that the foundation's hierarchy had about his stewardship. However, the motivation was more than purely self-preservation; the joint venture, which united the two leading agencies in the field, was, according to the immunoparasitologist, John David, truly original.

> There were mutual double-grants . . . in which the developed countries got money from [the RF] and the developing countries got funding from the TDR as a matching grant. It was wonderful: it was a way of getting expertise for the developing world and also using developing world people. It made for a very good collaboration, and was never done again.[97]

Alas, far from liberating Warren from his precarious standing with the Rockefeller trustees, according to Godal, their joint programme, further exacerbated the situation.

> There was a synergy between the GND and TDR and when I became Director in 1986, Ken invited me to go to his meetings and he suggested that we should partner, which I thought was a great idea. Then we could have both institutions in the North and institutions in the South. Because most of the TDR units were in the South, I suggested that the TDR should support the southern partners and Ken support the northern partners. And he agreed. But I think that marked the start of his end at the RF, because the board thought that Ken was consciously developing associations to support his friends [within the GND] but that was not the case.[98]

Warren's difficulties were a portent of the complicated relationship that Godal himself endured for a decade with the WHO's fourth Director-General Hiroshi Nakajima. From Nakajima, he received an education as to how the bureaucratic power game was a tangled exchange of horse-trading and backscratching. Likewise, Godal's dedication to health research priorities, health promotion and a belief in science made Nakajima feel uncomfortable. Alan Lopez worked at WHO for more than 20 years and has very little respect for Dr Nakajima: 'I had a hard time under Nakajima, and Tore had a difficult time as head of a scientific group that was well-respected outside of WHO, but under Nakajima, Tore suffered as well. Nakajima did all he could to neutralise us'.[99] During the Nakajima era, Godal developed the political survival skills that enabled him to protect TDR's ideals of equity and achieve decisive improvements against poverty causing diseases including the adoption of insecticide bed nets in malaria control, multi-drug treatment for leprosy and community-directed treatment with ivermectin for river blindness. Inevitably, there were painful defeats along the way, particularly the failure to persuade WHO's leadership to allow TDR to oversee the research component of the global TB programme. The 1980s and 1990s were turbulent decades, and with Geneva having the status of the Silicon Valley of global health, in a similar vein to high-technology corporations in California, the concept of mergers and acquisitions, or acquiring somebody else's turf, exercised minds. With the World Bank making large investments in TB studies in China, combined with Godal's desire to advance TB research globally, the time seemed right to bring tuberculosis into the TDR programme. However, it was not to be; the WHO bureaucracy won the day and Godal paid a heavy price, the friendship of Giorgio Torrigiani, who was WHO Director of the Division of Communicable Diseases. 'I remember once when I went to see Tore', Sue Tyrrell remembers,

> feeling anxious about something. Tore said, 'Sue, as my father would say, *you will have to learn to trust the system*'. However, the only time that I saw Tore down, was when he had worked really hard to get approval for TDR to take on TB, and the WHO leadership refused. Tore would defend the system, but I could see that sometimes the system gave him some knocks.[100]

By the early 1990s, Dr Nakajima's strong resistance to evidence-based medicine and the ideals of the World Bank's *World Development Report 1993*, clearly meant that the system had to be changed, and this is what Godal and like-minded colleagues set out to do. In the face of strong opposition from Dr Nakajima and senior WHO leadership, Godal, James Tulloch and Dean Jamison – together with other colleagues – established the highly influential WHO Ad Hoc Committee *'Investing in Health Research and Development'*, which reported in 1996. The report broke new ground in terms of developing research priority frameworks, assessment methods, cost-effectiveness research and Burden of Disease indicators. Importantly, no other WHO agency was advancing this critical agenda at the time, so the report filled a void and advocated the idea that health research and its application were essential to the development process. The report emphasised the continuing 'huge and unnecessary burden of infectious diseases among the poor that can be addressed with available cost-effective interventions. Addressing this unfinished agenda is mostly a matter of political will and (modest) commitment of resources'.[101] Acting as Co-Chair of the committee[102] was a decisive moment in Godal's life scientific, as it was a role that moved him out of TDR and into thinking more generally about research, while at the same time, strategically aligning him with a figure who had the 'political will' and intellectual strength to lead WHO into a new era. In 1998, Gro Harlem Brundtland became WHO Director-General. As a physician and former Chair of the Brundtland

Commission, she became an international leader in sustainable development and public health. Acting as Brundtland's adviser, Godal was able to use his worldwide tropical diseases network to aid his Norwegian friend navigate the future of global public health. With Brundtland's election as Director-General, the government of Norway, according to the former diplomat, Tarald Brautaset, 'decided to financially and diplomatically get behind health. Health became a priority, and the Norwegian aid budget was designed around health priorities identified by WHO, Gro Brundtland and Tore'.[103]

During the course of Godal's long career, a distinct pattern of behaviour emerges. He spends much time and intellectual effort building an institution, or a new organisation, or a global health strategy and once that undertaking is successful, he then passes the baton onto others and makes an orderly and uneventful departure. In this way, Godal is the agent of change, and then he relinquishes self-interest for the greater good. During his tenure, spending on programmes increased to 75% of resources, while staff numbers were reduced from 80 to 47. Godal also gave to TDR a new style of leadership character-ised by flat hierarchy, discussion and participation. In 1998, he left TDR after 12 years, to become the first director of Roll Back Malaria. In recognition of his work with TDR, in January 2000, Godal and Adetokunbo Lucas shared the Prince Mahidol Award from Thailand. A year later, Godal wrote a letter to the Armauer Hansen Research Institute, '[s]ince my international health career started at AHRI, I thought it would be appropriate to extend the benefit of the award to AHRI'. Accordingly, he donated the interest from his prize to be awarded as an annual Tore Godal Prize to young Ethiopian researchers who write papers on topics related to infectious diseases. Over the previous half century, a revolution had taken place. The AHRI marked the first real involve-ment of Norway in medical research in Africa. Bjørn Myrvang arrived in Addis Ababa in the autumn of 1969 and recognises the importance of Godal's contri-bution. 'Since Tore was the only person at the institute in the early days with research experience and international contacts, the success was mainly due to him'.[104] Today, the Armauer Hansen Research Institute is a centre of excellence in Africa, and globally, and highlights the development of low-income coun-tries and the necessary ownership of health.

Notes

1. K. Marx, *Capital*, vol. 1, chapter 7, "The Labour-Process and the Process of Pro-ducing Surplus-Value", section 1, "The Labour-Process or the Production of Use-Values".
2. T. Godal, "Auto-immunity of the thyroid: On the etiology and effect of thyroglobu-lin antibodies", PhD thesis, University of Oslo, 1967.
3. A. Crump, "Tore Godal: Pragmatic opportunist championing global public health", *Trends in Parasitology*, August 2006, 22 (8), pp. 378–384.
4. Interview with Tore Godal, August 2018.

5. Interview with Helga Fogstad, June 2020.
6. Tore Godal's mother, together with her sister who was a nurse, wrote and produced *The Cabbage* newsletter for the local Lutheran church that among other things, gave horticultural advice about how to grow vegetables, and recipes for potato dishes.
7. He was nominated for the Nobel Prize in Literature in 1919, 1925, 1929 and again in 1932.
8. S. K. Sarker, *William Wordsworth: A Companion* (New Delhi: Atlantic, 2003), pp. 150–152.
9. The impact of the Nazi occupation on Norwegian society was especially deep. In trials that lasted from 1945 until 1957, more than 90,000 cases of collaboration were investigated and 46,000 people were sentenced. Far from stabilising the country, as the returning government-in-exile had hoped, the trials had a profoundly polarising effect. This was the most expansive judicial reckoning anywhere in post-war Europe.
10. Interview with Helga Fogstad, June 2020.
11. A. M. Silverstein, "The curious case of the 1960 Nobel Prize to Burnet and Medawar", *Immunology*, 2016, 147 (3), pp. 269–274.
12. Interview with James Gowan, August 2013.
13. J. L. Gowans, "The recirculation of lymphocytes from blood to lymph in the rat", *Journal of Physiology*, 1959, 146, pp. 54–69.
14. T. Gould, *Don't Fence Me In: From the Curse to Cure Leprosy in Modern Times* (London: Bloomsbury, 2005), p. 37.
15. G. A. Hansen, "Undersoglser angaende spedalskhedens arsager", *Norsk Magastin for Laegevitenskapen*, 1874, 4 (1). For an English version of this major work, see G. A. Hansen, C. Looft, (transl. N. Walker), *Leprosy: In Its Clinical and Pathological Aspects* (Bristol: John Wright & Co, 1895 – reprinted in 1973), p. 162.
16. Medical Research Council, Streptomycin in Tuberculosis trials committee, "Streptomycin treatment for pulmonary tuberculosis", *British Medical Journal*, 1948, 2, pp. 749–782.
17. E. M. Tansey, "Philip Montagu D'Arcy Hart (1900–2006)", *Journal of the Royal Society of Medicine*, 2006, 99, pp. 535–539.
18. Hart, together with among others, Richard Doll, Martin Roff and Julian Tudor Hard were members of the Sigerist Society that met between 1947 and 1955. Sigerist envisioned a society in which the benefits of medical science would be for the benefit of all and not just for the rich who could afford to pay for health care.
19. C. Keating, *Smoking Kills: The Revolutionary Life of Richard Doll* (Oxford: Signal Books, 2009), p. 82.
20. Interview with Bjørn Myrvang, February 2021.
21. A. Crump, "Tore Godal: Pragmatic opportunist championing global public health", *Trends in Parasitology*, 2006, 22 (8), p. 379.
22. B. Myrvang, T. Godal, D. S. Samuel, S. S. Frøland, Y. K. Song, "Immune responsiveness to *Mycobacterium leprae* and other mycobacterial antigens throughout the clinical and histopathological spectrum of leprosy", *Clinical and Experimental Immunology*, 1973, 14, pp. 541–553.
23. Interview with Bjørn Myrvang, February 2021.
24. T. Gould, *Don't Fence Me In: From the Curse to Cure Leprosy in Modern Times* (London: Bloomsbury, 2005), p. 56.
25. Interview with Bjørn Myrvang, February 2021.
26. T. Godal, B. Myrvang, R. D. Samuel, W. F. Ross, M. Løfgren, "Mechanism of 'reactions' in borderline tuberculoid (BT) leprosy. A preliminary report", *Acta Pathologica et Microbiologica Scandinavica. Section A*, 1973 (Suppl. 236), pp. 45–53.

27. T. Godal, B. Myklestad, D. R. Samuel, B. Myrvang, "Characterization of the cellular immune defect in lepraomatous leprosy: A specific lack of circulating *Mycobacerium leprae*-reactive lymphocytes", *Clinical and Experimental Immunology*, 1971, 9, pp. 821–831.
28. Interview with Tore Godal, August 2018.
29. Barry Bloom email communication, March 2021.
30. Godal and his colleagues found that patients "responded quite well to the BCG."
31. A. Crump, "Tore Godal: Pragmatic opportunist championing global public health", *Trends in Parasitology*, 2006, 22 (8), p. 379.
32. 1974 WHA27.52.
33. A. Snyder, "Obituary: Halfdan Mahler", *Lancet*, 7 January 2017, 389 (10064), p. 30.
34. World Health Organization, *Twelfth Programme Report of the UNDP/World Bank/WHO Special Programme for Research and Training in Tropical Diseases (TDR)*, (1995), p. 1.
35. World Health Organization, *Twelfth Programme Report of the UNDP/World Bank/WHO Special Programme for Research and Training in Tropical Diseases (TDR)*, (1995), p. 9.
36. Interview with Bjørn Myrvang, February 2021.
37. Interview with Barry Bloom, October 2020.
38. This was a time of innovation, and in 1971, Margaret Snyder, the founding director of the Voluntary Fund for the Decade for Women, which later became known as Unifem, started working for the United Nations in Addis Ababa, on programmes for African women centred on healthcare and support for children. As an expert on establishing voluntary organisations, Snyder helped to set up a programme at the UN Economic Commission for Africa (ECA) to support women in their roles as farmers, entrepreneurs and often the main family breadwinners. It evolved into the African Training and Research Centre for Women (ATRCW).
39. T. Gould, *Don't Fence Me In: From the Curse to Cure Leprosy in Modern Times* (London: Bloomsbury, 2005), p. 325.
40. Interview with Helga Fogstad, June 2020.
41. T. Godal, B. Myrvang, D. R. Samuel, W. F. Ross, M. Løfgren, "Mechanism of 'reactions' in borderline tuberculoid (BT) leprosy. A preliminary report", *Acta Pathologica et Microbiologica Scandinavica. Section A*, 1973 (Suppl. 236), p. 45.
42. World Health Organization, *Twelfth Programme Report of the UNDP/World Bank/WHO Special Programme for Research and Training in Tropical Diseases (TDR)*, (1995), p. 9.
43. World Health Organization, *Twelfth Programme Report of the UNDP/World Bank/WHO Special Programme for Research and Training in Tropical Diseases (TDR)*, (1995), p. 7.
44. There was a lot of resentment from the relevant disease control divisions in WHO – the Malaria Action Programme, the Parasitic Diseases Programme, and Vector Biology and Control Programme. Their preference was for the donors to give money to expand their well-established research programmes instead of creating a new entity.
45. WHO originally planned to establish a research institute in Ndola, Zambia that would serve as the nerve centre of the new programme. Following Halfdan Mahler's election as director-general in 1973, his deputy, Professor T. Adeoye, Lambo, a Nigerian specialist in psychiatry took responsibility for the new tropical disease research initiative. He became convinced that Ndola, a copper mining town close to the border with the DRC, would become the centre of excellence in biomedical research. His conviction was further galvanised when President Kaunda offered two floors of a new hospital building in Ndola to accommodate the new research

initiative. However, it was during a site visit to Zambia that Sune Bergstrom decided to alter the TDR operational strategy from an institution-based programme to a networking construct. Bergstrom became increasingly convinced that the idea to create a mini-replica of the US-based National Institutes of Health in a geographically remote part of Zambia was ill conceived.

46. Interview with Tore Godal, August 2018.
47. Interview with Tore Godal, August 2018.
48. W. F. Kirchheimer, E. E. Storrs, "Attempts to establish the armadillo (*Dasypus novemcinctus* Linn) as a model for the study of leprosy", *International Journal of Leprosy*, 1971, 39, p. 369.
49. R. R. Young, V. Mehra, T. Sweetser, T. M. Buchanan, J. Clark-Curtiss, R. W. Davis, B. R. Bloom, "Genes for the major protein of *Mycobacterium leprae*", *Nature*, 1985, 316, p. 450.
50. World Health Organization, *Twelfth Programme Report of the UNDP/World Bank/ WHO Special Programme for Research and Training in Tropical Diseases (TDR)*, (1995), p. 4.
51. C. Keating, "The genesis of the Global Burden of Disease Study", *Lancet*, 2018, 391 (10137), pp. 2316–2317.
52. Interview with Chris Murray, April 2021.
53. K. S. Warren, C. C. Jimenez (eds.), *The Great Neglected Diseases of Mankind Biomedical Research Network: 1978–1988* (New York: The Rockefeller Foundation, 1988), p. 1.
54. D. H. Molyneu, A. Asamoa-Bah, A. Fenwick, L. Savioli, P. Hotez, "The history of the neglected tropical disease movement", *Transactions of the Royal Society of Tropical Medicine & Hygiene*, 2021, 115, pp. 169–175.
55. C. Keating, *Kenneth Warren and the Great Neglected Diseases of Mankind Programme: The Transformation of Geographical Medicine in the US and Beyond* (New York: Springer, 2017).
56. K. S. Warren, "The difficult art, science, and politics of setting health priorities", *Lancet*, 27 August 1988, pp. 498–499.
57. S. Halstead, J. Walsh, K. Warren (eds.), *Good Health at Low Cost* (Bellagio and New York: Rockefeller Foundation, 1985).
58. Interview with Sir Richard Peto, July 2018.
59. Interview with Sir Gustav Nossal, November 2018.
60. A. O. Lucas, *It Was the Best of Times: From Local to Global Health* (Ibadan, Nigeria: BookBuilders, 2010), p. 202.
61. Interview with Tore Godal, August 2018.
62. R. Lane, "Tore Godal: Quiet colossus of global health", *Lancet*, 25 November 2019, 394 (10215), p. 2142.
63. T. Godal, S. Fenderud, "Human B-cell neoplasms in relation to normal B-cell differentiation and maturation processes", *Advances in Cancer Research*, 1982, 36, pp. 211–255.
64. T. Godal, "Immunological aspects of leprosy: Present status", *Progress in Allergy*, 1978, 25, pp. 211–242.
65. Interview with Bill Foege, March 2020.
66. B. R. Bloom, T. Godal, "Selective primary health care: Strategies for control of disease in the developing world. V. Leprosy", *Reviews of Infectious Diseases*, 1983, 5 (4), pp. 765–780.
67. Interview with Helga Fogstad, June 2020.
68. World Health Organization, *Twelfth Programme Report of the UNDP/World Bank/ WHO Special Programme for Research and Training in Tropical Diseases (TDR)*, (1995), p. 19.

69. G. Watts, "Obituary adetokunbo O. Lucas", *The Lancet*, 30 January 2021, 397, p. 368.
70. Interview with Helga Fogstad, June 2020.
71. T. Godal, "Fighting the parasites of poverty: Public research, private industry, and tropical diseases", *Science*, 1994, 264 (5167), pp. 1864–1866.
72. T. Godal, "Fighting the parasites of poverty: Public research, private industry, and tropical diseases", *Science*, 1994, 264 (5167), p. 1865.
73. Interview with Tore Godal, August 2018.
74. A. O. Lucas, *It Was the Best of Times: From Local to Global Health* (Ibadan, Nigeria: BookBuilders, 2010), p. 150.
75. Interview with Sue Tyrrell, April 2021.
76. Interview with David Evans, April 2021.
77. A. Crump, "Tore Godal: Pragmatic opportunist championing global public health", *Trends in Parasitology*, 2006, 22 (8), p. 379.
78. Interview with David Evans, April 2021.
79. Personal communication email from Alan Fairlamb, February 2021.
80. Personal communication email from Brian Greenwood, May 2021.
81. Interview with Tore Godal, August 2018.
82. A. Crump, "Tore Godal: Pragmatic opportunist championing global public health", *Trends in Parasitology*, 2006, 22 (8), p. 381.
83. Personal communication email from Bridget Ogilvie, April 2020.
84. Personal communication email from Brian Greenwood, April 2020.
85. Interview with Tore Godal, August 2018.
86. Interview with Lisa Jacobs, November 2020.
87. Interview with David Evans, April 2021.
88. Interview with Barry Bloom, October 2020.
89. Interview with David Evans, April 2021.
90. T. Godal, "Opinion: Do we have the architecture for health aid right? Increasing global aid effectiveness", *Nature Reviews, Microbiology*, 2005, 3 (11), pp. 899–903.
91. Interview with Sue Tyrrell, April 2021.
92. Interview with Barry Bloom, October 2020.
93. A. Boseley, "Norway's Prime Minister Jens Stoltenberg: Leader on MDG4", *Profile, Lancet*, 22 September 2007, 370, p. 1027.
94. Interview with Chris Murray, April 2021.
95. Interview with Barry Bloom, October 2020.
96. "The TDR-Rockefeller Foundation joint funding venture, announced last year, was seen as an important way to strengthen collaboration between different groups of research workers – to be backed by substantial R&D support. Over 200 'letters of intent' were submitted, and, of these, 29 have been invited to prepare formal proposals – although possibly no more than 10 will be selected for major funding." *Parasitology Today*, 1988, 4 (5), p. 123.
97. C. Keating, *Kenneth Warren and the Great Neglected Diseases of Mankind Programme: The Transformation of Geographical Medicine in the US and Beyond* (New York: Springer, 2017), p. 110.
98. C. Keating, *Kenneth Warren and the Great Neglected Diseases of Mankind Programme: The Transformation of Geographical Medicine in the US and Beyond* (New York: Springer, 2017), p. 110.
99. Interview with Alan Lopez, August 2020.
100. Interview with Sue Tyrrell, March 2021.
101. Ad Hoc Committee on Health Research Relating to Future Intervention Options, *Summary of Investing in Health Research and Development* (Geneva: World Health Organization, 1996) (Document TDR/GEN/96.2.), 6.

102. The committee brought together an influential group of people who played an important role in global health over the coming decades. The Ad Hoc members included among others Seth Berkeley, Chris Murray, Alan Lopez, Susanna Sans, Baron Paul Janssen, Derek Yach, Julio Frenk, and Richard Peto.
103. Interview with Tarald Brautaset, August 2020.
104. Interview with Bjørn Myrvang, February 2021.

2 River Blindness and the Ivermectin Story

The story of ivermectin is a reminder of the power of research.

Donald Bundy[1]

The prevention and cure of river blindness is one of the most remarkable stories in medical history. It depended upon scientific ingenuity, Pharmaco-Philanthropy, innovative public–private partnerships, good will and persistence. This is the story of how a successful coalition in global health forms a decisive moment in the history of understanding, preventing and curing a human disease. In the middle of the last century, it was estimated that about five million square miles of the earth's surface, and some 20 million people, were infected with river blindness (*onchocerciasis*), a chronically disabling condition which affected the poor in many lower-income countries.[2] The parasitic disease, caused by the filarial threadworm *Onchocerca volvulus*, is transmitted through the infected bite of blackflies of the genus *Simulium*, which inhabit fast-flowing streams and rivers. Blackflies are vectors for the parasites, which burrow into the skin and grow into mature worms, sometimes measuring more than 60 centimetres, or two feet, in length. Adult worms develop in subcutaneous nodules where the females produce larvae, which migrate as microfilariae into surrounding tissue and the eyes. During this migration, the human host experiences intense, unbearable itching, which can lead to devastating dermatological diseases, stigma, social isolation, reduced economic performance and irreversible blindness.[3] An adult worm can live for up to 16 years in the human body,[4] and the fear of impending blindness, combined with the blackflies' unremitting biting intensity, led in some parts of the savannah areas of West Africa to the abandonment of human settlements on fecund lands near rivers. The physical suffering and economic desolation caused by this insidious disease was such that strategies evolved to help reduce the inexorable sequence of exposure, disability and penury.

DOI: 10.4324/9781003363859-3

During the colonial era, European researchers developed theories to explain the transmission of the disease, its epidemiology and a method for its control. In 1930, the Belgian ophthalmologist Jean Hissette, working in the Belgian Congo (now Zaire), published a short article in which he described the lesions caused by the microfilariae and geographically identified the locations of isolated villages where large numbers of men had been blinded by the disease.[5] In the following decade, the British ophthalmologist Harold Ridley carried out important research in the north-west of the Gold Coast (now Ghana), drawing attention to the manifestations of the disease in the retina.[6] Their joint contribution to the description of retinal damage and onchocercal blindness was eponymously recognised, and is now known as the Hissette-Ridley fundus. At the time, in the absence of a safe and effective drug with which to treat the disease, entomologists put forward the idea of vector elimination as a means of controlling the infection. Encouragingly, the British had developed sophisticated entomological expertise through their attempts to reduce tsetse fly populations as a means of preventing African sleeping sickness. Building on this tradition, the entomologist J.P. McMahon succeeded in eradicating blackflies in the Kodera Valley, Kenya, by treating the streams with DDT.[7] Although this pioneering work took place in the ominously named Valley of the Blind, the indigenous *Simulium neavei*, which only laid its eggs on the bodies of freshwater crabs (*potamonautes niloticus*), was a less adaptable vector than the West African *S. damnosum*, which had a considerable flight range, and laid its eggs on plentiful vegetation in rivers. Historically, however, this was a telling experiment, and the eradication of the disease from the Kodera Valley inspired several vector control projects in West Africa in the 1950s and 1960s. Yet the ability to control the blackfly vector was tempered by the knowledge that adult worms could live in humans for ten to 15 years. Consequently, vector control to break the human-fly-human cycle would need to be sustained until the adult parasites had died of natural causes, demanding a programme lasting 15 or more years.[8]

The combined influence of the vector control experiments, together with a serendipitous meeting between the French evangelical entomologist René Le Berre and the President of the World Bank, Robert McNamara, transformed river blindness from being a peripheral disease with little or no political voice, to one of pre-eminence in the world of neglected tropical diseases (NTDs). Le Berre, an advocate of spraying insecticide on blackfly breeding grounds to kill the larvae and prevent onchocerciasis from spreading, persuaded McNamara to visit Upper Volta (now Burkina Faso) to see at first hand the human cost exacted by the disease. On this expedition, McNamara visited a village on the banks of the White Volta River where the disease affected more than three-quarters of the population and more than 12% of the villagers were blind. According to one of Le Berre's obituary notices, he adapted the phrase 'villages at the end of the road' to express the isolation and lack of support for these communities.[9] The sight of abandoned villages in fertile valleys deepened this dystopian health picture further, at a time of severe drought in sub-Saharan Africa. This shocked McNamara, and the experience marked a historic moment in both the guiding philosophy of the World Bank and the natural history of onchocerciasis in Africa and across the globe. McNamara brought the necessary political persuasion to the ideal of seeing health as an investment, not simply an expenditure. Accordingly, when he returned to report to his Board in Washington, DC, he persuaded the World Bank to start investing in disease control as a means of alleviating poverty. The conversion of McNamara foreshadowed a sequence of events that led to new political and financial support for an unprecedented aerial vector control programme, bringing together the World Bank and the WHO. For Bjorn Thylefors, a Swedish tropical ophthalmologist working in the Algerian Sahara at the time, this moment was defining:

> I'm sorry to say it, but we needed an economist and the former US Defence Secretary to tell us this obvious thing, which the World Health Organisation (WHO) had not particularly thought of. WHO was treating disease; they didn't see it in a bigger context of community development, society development and economy.[10]

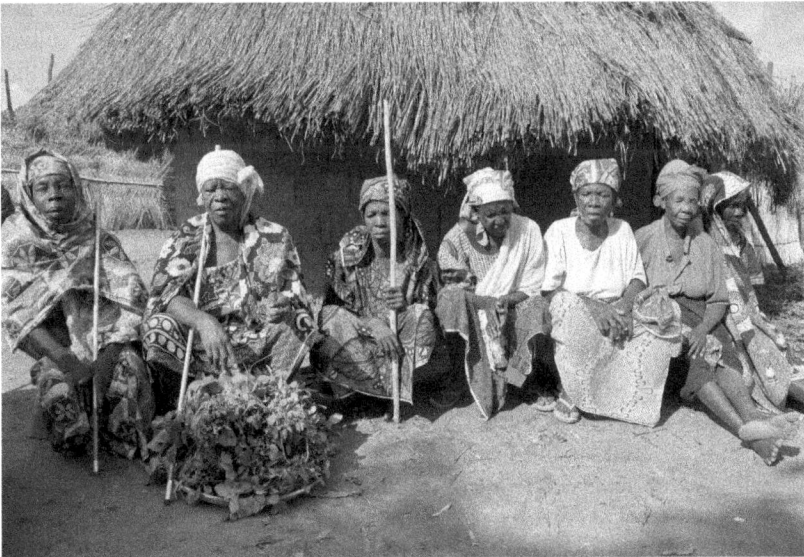

Figure 2.1   Seven Nigerian women farmers blinded by onchocerciasis. In 2007, they were gathered together to receive ivermectin tablets at a central distribution point.

Source: Courtesy of Andy Crump.

The Onchocerciasis Control Programme for West Africa (OCP)

The prevention of blindness was the main clinical reason for initiating the Onchocerciasis Control Programme (OCP) in West Africa in 1974. The OCP was a significant undertaking in a number of ways. It created a joint mission between the WHO and the World Bank; the first occasion that the latter had become directly involved in health issues. By establishing itself in Ouagadougou, the capital of Burkina Faso, the OCP helped to make the city the centre of the onchocerciasis universe for the next 40 years. This placed onchocerciasis on the global political map, which tangentially had the effect of separating the disease from other neglected tropical diseases (NTDs), including trachoma, an even more pervasive cause of blindness in the developing world.[11] The programme encompassed a vast geographical area, initially operating in seven countries, before expanding to 11 states in the savannah areas of West Africa. Aerial operations using both helicopters and fixed-wing aircraft started in January 1975, with the programme based entirely on vector control with larvicides to prevent the transmission of river blindness.

Since the publication of Rachel Carson's prescient book *Silent Spring* in 1962, which showed that pesticides did in fact damage birds' eggshells, there had been concern about the environmental damage caused by insecticides, and therefore, the OCP programme was under constant scrutiny by an independent monitoring unit.[12] OCP was very successful, however, in protecting communities in the worst known areas of the disease, reducing poverty and increasing arable production by enabling previously abandoned land to be brought back into cultivation. Its efficacy was costly though, with expenditure reaching almost one billion US dollars over the programme's 27-year history.[13] Moreover, the OCP strategy that had been so successfully deployed in West Africa could not be transferred to other countries across the continent, where larger populations of infected individuals lived with insufferable itching, concomitant social isolation and were at risk of losing their vision. Both epidemiologically and ecologically, the OCP had reached the limits of its geographical frontiers and utility. Any expansion of the programme's operations faced insurmountable difficulties, as succinctly explained by the Togolese medical entomologist Azodoga Seketeli, who joined OCP in March 1976:

> Flies don't know borders – they can fly over 400 kilometres from their breeding site. . . . But should international communities have been prepared to finance vector control operations throughout Africa where onchocerciasis is prevalent? Technically, for us entomologists, it would not have been possible to do. Many rivers were completely hidden under canopies of forests, so we would be putting insecticide on the leaves of the trees instead of into the water. We couldn't have done it technically – no way.[14]

Clearly if the OCP could not expand to prevent the people of Central and East Africa suffering from the devastating effects of river blindness, another remedy had to be sought.

The Play of Chance and the Path of Discovery

In 1945, Harold Ridley had recognised the increasing potential of modern science to provide new means of treatment and prevention of tropical diseases and made this prophetic statement: 'Many preparations already produced await trials and it is inconceivable that in the end science will be defeated by a filarial'.[15] Ridley's prediction that perhaps valuable treatments already existed yet lay undiscovered highlighted the role of luck and the play of chance that is so often decisive in medical innovation. The classic example is Alexander Fleming's serendipitous discovery of a mysterious mould in a Petri dish that eventually led to the thera-peutic discovery of penicillin by scientists in Oxford in 1941. A similar chance event was to have a transformative effect on the clinical management of river blindness. In the early 1970s, the US pharmaceutical company Merck began col-laborating with the Kitasato Institute in Japan. The Institute's role was to select soil microorganisms that might be the source of active chemicals and send them to Merck's laboratories in Rahway, New Jersey, for anti-parasite testing.[16] Many tens of thousands of isolates were analysed but no 'magic bullet', to adapt Paul Ehr-lich's phrase, was forthcoming. However, the sequence of unending failure was dramatically altered when Satoshi Omura's group sent soil sample No.OS3153, taken from the thirteenth fairway of a Japanese golf course, to William 'Bill' Campbell, Merck's Director of Basic Parasitology.[17] From this extreme chance event, Campbell and his team developed the drug ivermectin, a broad-spectrum anti-parasitic drug. In addition to the obvious health benefits of the discovery, the breakthrough led to a pioneering drug donation programme that inaugurated a new technique of treating parasitic infection, and to Campbell and Omura win-ning the 2015 Nobel Prize for their role in transforming global health.[18]

Campbell had joined Ashton Cutler's parasitology group at Merck in 1957 with some reservations:

> I imagined that my destiny would be an academic teacher-researcher at a uni-versity, but after meeting Cutler it seemed like [working for Merck] would be fun, attractive and appealing work. I had grave misgivings because [Merck] was a corporation, a for-profit outfit, but it just turned out much better than I expected.[19]

Campbell joined Merck's burgeoning animal health research division and forged his career in their anti-helminthic programme. There he divided his time between veterinary research and human parasitology, spending seven years working on treatments for schistosomiasis but without any success. Conterminously, on one of his early research visits to South America to study Chagas disease, Campbell had even drafted a memo on onchocerciasis, indicating a long-standing interest in the disease. Moreover, he was steadfast in his belief that almost without exception, 'in terms of infectious diseases, all parasitic drugs have been developed empirically, by ancient clinical observation, trial and error, but [ultimately] empirically'.[20]

Following the practices of the Oxford-based biochemical scientists who had isolated penicillin for clinical use, Campbell deployed fermentation techniques and the use of mice in his attempts to find a new potent drug with anti-parasitic properties. The mice were infected by two different parasites (a coccidian and a nematode) and then given food, which had been impregnated with a crude broth containing the isolated fungus. The accurate testing of thousands of soil samples on the animals was made possible by the application of an innovative 'tandem assay' system, assiduously monitored by a dedicated team of technicians and laboratory scientists. In 1975, as part of the ongoing test of samples sent from the Kitasato Institute, 54 infected mice were given food infused with a fermented broth containing bacteria. At the end of the experiment, *one* of the mice, which had been treated with the fungus OS3153, isolated from a Japanese golf course, was found to be free of nematode infection. The extraordinary organism *Streptomyces avermitilis* had been discovered – and constitutes the chemical base of ivermectin. Even though the search for more soil samples continued across the globe, no other organism producing a molecule with similar anti-parasitic properties was found.[21] Incredibly, nature had selectively evolved the fungus from the material universe to produce a molecule that was safe to use across species, including dogs, horses, fish and humans, and that was effective against roundworm parasites and many arthropod parasites. Within weeks, Campbell and his team had produced a variety of chemical compounds for use in veterinary medicine, including a dog heartworm drug that made Merck the most financially successful animal health company in corporate history. In fact, so great is Campbell's association with this filarial worm that when President Obama honoured the 2015 Nobel Prize winner at a ceremony in the White House, he presented the delighted parasitologist with a white knitted wool imitation of the heartworm.[22]

What guided Campbell and his team in their work by a singular objective – to make good medicines.[23] Yet, as many applied biomedical researchers will testify, drug discovery is an inexact science. In the era of monoclonal antibodies, molecular biology and genomic inventiveness, the methodological approach deployed differs greatly from the empirical screening process used to discover ivermectin. Essentially, the emphasis today is on seeking to understand basic biochemistry and cell biology, to identify a difference between the parasite metabolism and that of the host, and to exploit that pathway to develop a drug that is harmful to the parasite and harmless to the host. For Campbell, the inexorable rise of modern translational medicine has seen an unfortunate corresponding decline in the status of the scientific techniques that he and his colleagues perfected:

> My belief is that we know how to discover new anti-infectious drugs unpredictably, we do not know how to discover them predictably. Nevertheless, today people want to control drug discovery and so have abandoned empirical approaches. We [need] to do both kinds of research, but it was a great mistake to abandon the ways that worked. The empirical method has been tainted by its simplicity.[24]

Ivermectin (brand name Mectizan®) was isolated from nature, and its detection shows that on occasion, medical advance depends on adapting to human needs the solutions that nature has already found. If the discovery of the drug required persistence, dedication and enlightened strategic thinking, so too did its future development as the panacea for human onchocerciasis. This process was to underscore the indispensable role of scientific management in securing funds and making judgements on the direction of research programmes, and it emphasises the defining role of one individual in shaping the trajectory of an infectious disease.

The Mectizan Donation Programme

Roy Vagelos, a chemist, physician, and head of the Merck Research Laboratories, had been closely following the exciting progress of the ivermectin's development as an anthelmintic drug. In 1978, evidence suggested that the drug was effective against microfilariae of *Onchocerca cervicalise* in horses, which belonged to the same genus that caused river blindness in humans.[25] When Vagelos heard of this discovery, he encouraged Campbell to expand the search for human therapeutic uses.[26] Campbell, the quintessential experimenter, believes that the subsequent clinical trials conducted by his Merck colleague Mohammed Aziz, in Senegal and Ghana, with the help of the WHO Special Programme for Research and Training in Tropical Diseases (TDR) were the telling experiments.[27] TDR's mandate was to discover and develop new and improved technologies for the control of tropical diseases affecting the poor in developing countries.[28] The study, on a small number of lightly infected people, established that a single ivermectin tablet, taken once a year, was effective against the microfilariae that lived in the eyes and skin, without provoking any severe side effects.[29] While it appeared to be something of a wonder drug, ivermectin was not perfect. As a suppressor drug with a high potency, it destroyed the larvae (microfilariae), but it was not fatal to the adult worm inside the human host. Thus, a programme of control would necessitate long-term annual treatments involving much expense and complex logistical planning (until the death of the adult worms after 15 years). This compelling evidence presented Merck with a moral conundrum. How could they balance their corporate obligation to make profits from a drug that was too expensive for a population of the world's poorest people to buy? It appeared that the company had entangled itself in a business paradox: the development of an effective therapeutic for patients too poor to afford the treatment.

As an established behemoth of the pharmaceutical industry, and unmistakably a 'for profit outfit',[30] nevertheless, the company had established a tradition of benevolence. After WWII, George Merck had given Japan access to the antibiotic streptomycin, by granting free licences to two Japanese pharmaceutical companies to manufacture the drug for the treatment of tuberculosis. Vagelos built upon this philanthropic tradition in a stunning gesture of corporate generosity that marked the beginning of a successful coalition in global health. At the time, the infrastructure to get aid to 'the villages at the end of the road' was not yet in place; there seemed no way round the bureaucratic quagmire of the WHO, and Merck's search for a co-sponsor of their river blindness research had proved unrewarding. Vagelos, an imposing leader with a formidable presence and strong opinions, felt no divided loyalty between corporate stewardship and social need; as head of the company, he decided that the only way out of the impasse was to donate the drug free to those who couldn't pay, vowing to donate as much as was needed, for a long as was needed. He came to his decision free from any moral ambiguity:

> There were no alternatives. The drug was not going to be used unless someone made it available. And I knew the company could afford it because it was growing at the time. You have to do what's right at the time, and for that moment and this population of people that was the right thing to do. My major responsibility was drug discovery and getting it to the people.[31]

The important decision to donate ivermectin is starkly revealed by Adetokunbo O. Lucas, the then Director of TDR. In his autobiography, Lucas describes a meeting held at Merck to discuss the worrying question of the price of the drug.

> We were received by Dr Roy Vagelos, the chief executive officer of the company. He put us at ease with a warm welcome. He prepared and served me a nice cup of coffee – an experience I intend to mention to my grandchildren. I was well prepared for tough negotiations about the pricing of the drug. I had made notes about WHO/TDR's contributions both in kind and in cash for screening the drug and for conducting clinical trials in Ghana and in Nigeria. I had rehearsed my speech about the significance of the partnership between WHO/TDR and the company, a shared goal with contributions from both sides. Then came the bombshell! Roy Vagelos told us, in confidence, of the corporate decision to donate the drug . . . Such a generous gesture was unprecedented.[32]

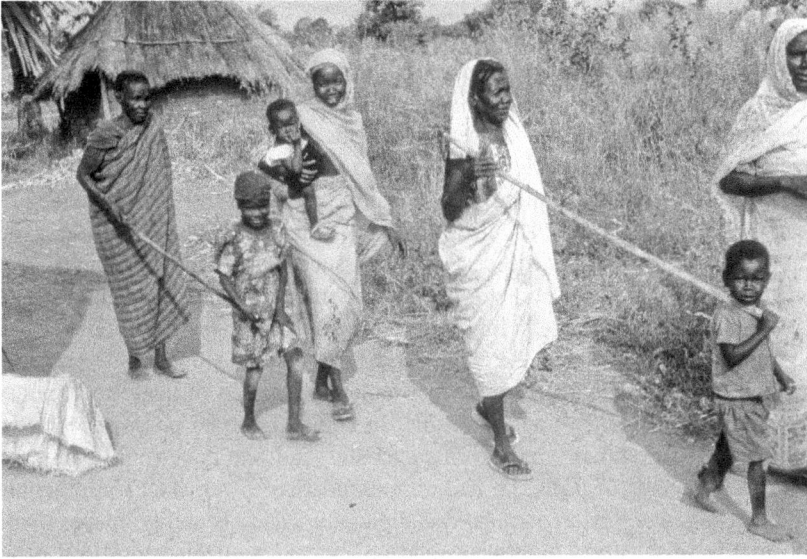

Figure 2.2 Children leading blind adults in Sudan, in 1997. Traditionally, sighted children were called upon to lead their blind parents and relatives.

Source: Courtesy of Andy Crump.

Meanwhile, for those caring for river blindness patients in the field, the donation was universally welcomed. Bjorn Thylefors viewed the decision as being made in the spirit of their chosen profession of healing: 'Vagelos was a physician after all. He had a heart. He was not a lawyer, and he really had the vision. It was a very brave decision, and it was really a fantastic thing'.[33] The donation transcended financial imperatives and had a profound impact on the treatment of river blindness. In order for this to be achieved however, some initial obstacles had to be overcome. When Merck first started looking for an institution to head up the donation programme, no one quite knew how it would work, as this was the first time that a free donation on such an unprecedented scale had taken place. Moreover, Merck's eventual offer to WHO to produce the donated molecule under licence, and to run the programme, came at a time when there was widespread suspicion of pharmaceutical companies. Another obstacle to acceptance was the formidable Halfdan Mahler, Director-General of WHO. Mahler had been shaken by the collapse of the WHO's malaria eradication programmes in the 1970s, and this influenced his subsequent thinking.[34] As a physician, Mahler had trained in public health, specialising in tuberculosis, and had then worked on mass campaigns in South America and India that he had come to dislike.[35] Both ethically and philosophically, he viewed the status quo as being untenable, noting that there was clear evidence that 'the scientific and technical structures of public health are crumbling'.[36] For Mahler, the solution was not science and a selective so-called 'vertical' approach, but a doctrine of comprehensive primary health care.[37] In addition to methodological differences, Mahler also disliked the corporate sector and the concept of making profits from human medicines. Therefore, WHO rejected Merck's offer to oversee the donation of the drug.

This was the delicate equipoise, which foreshadowed a meeting attended by Tore Godal in October 1986, held at Merck's headquarters in Rahway, New Jersey. Just a few months earlier, Godal had succeeded the Nigerian physician Adetokunbo O. Lucas as Director of TDR, an institution that had demonstrated a willingness to participate in innovative forms of public–private collaborations for tropical disease drug development. Godal was determined to use his powerful position in global health to reduce the intolerable burden of neglected tropical diseases on the world's poorest people. In addition, Godal possessed another important and eventually telling characteristic, and one that would define his tenure as Director of TDR; he had a determination to turn ideas into actions that were positive.[38] Moreover, he was diplomatic, and his ability to speak with equanimity to scientists, politicians and policymakers enabled him to become a powerful advocate for global health. Above all, he valued honesty, reliability and trust. To Godal, 'trust is the basis of everything in global health. Your word *is* your word'.[39] Intrinsically, he knew that development was impossible without trust, and it exerted a powerful influence over him throughout his life. As we shall see, this attitude enabled Godal not only to have been present at many of the decisive moments in global health, but instrumental in making them happen.[40] Also attending the meeting at Merck's headquarters with Godal was the Gambian physician Ebrahim Samba, Director of OCP, and Nyle Brady, a senior administrator at the United States Agency for International Aid (USAID), one of the largest institutions of its kind in the world. Three months previously, Adetokunbo Lucas had secured a preliminary commitment from Merck to give the drug free but there was still a lot of opposition – both within the company and at WHO. After a cordial welcome, Roy Vagelos turned to Nyle Brady and asked if USAID would subsidise the use of ivermectin in poorer countries. When Nyle Brady answered 'no', Roy Vagelos announced to everyone in the room: 'Then we will make it available gratis'.[41] This was a decisive and memorable moment for Godal, 'I remember the words exactly, because "gratis" is used in Norwegian too'.[42] The Merck negotiations reinforced his conviction of the need for equitable and comprehensive collaborations between the private and public sectors.[43] Intuitively, Godal understood what this donation could mean for the control of the disease. Speed was of the essence, and when the meeting ended, he flew directly to Geneva to brief his TDR colleagues and began to consider how to accelerate the delivery of ivermectin to those communities most in need.

Paradoxically, three senior WHO officials then approached Godal and tried to persuade him not to accept the donation as it would set a difficult precedent for other drug manufacturers. Godal suspected that they had been lobbied by the pharmaceutical industry that it was not right that a medicament should be free of charge. 'But I said, "are you crazy? To throw away your negotiation cards before the negotiation?"'[44] A decade earlier, while attempting to promote a leprosy vaccine, Godal had learned that it was possible to set up large-scale international trials and run and evaluate them in low-income countries. This was the approach TDR utilised to prove that ivermectin was a safe microfilaricide. TDR's involvement in river blindness increased substantially with the start of trials of the effectiveness of ivermectin in community treatments programmes in 1987. Thirteen community-based trials were conducted between 1987 and 1989, and over 120,000 individual doses of ivermectin were given. As the historian Michael R. Reich has written,

> Of the 13 community trials, TDR funded five studies in Liberia, Cameroon, Malawi, Guatemala, and Nigeria and spent $2.35 million. . . . This substantial financial commitment by TDR shows its strong concern about the implications of ivermectin for onchocerciasis control programmes.[45]

Trust is the glue that holds coalitions together, and if a control programme would require Mectizan® to be given to many millions of people, then everyone had to have faith in its safety and efficacy. During the early years of being Director of TDR Godal learned some valuable lessons. First, the need to create and sustain an atmosphere of confidence in the bureaucracy. Second, tempo is crucial when starting a programme, because the forces of opposition, 'those who want to hold you down, they always move more slowly – so you must be positive and have the speed to stay ahead of them'.[46]

Just months after the meeting at Merck's headquarters, an onchocerciasis scientific conference took place in Ouagadougou, which presented Godal with the opportunity to discuss the ivermectin donation with colleagues, and then to embark upon site visits to TDR-supported fieldworkers across Africa. Alas, after swimming in a pool with adulterated water, Godal was 'stricken'[47] with a severe case of Hepatitis A-non B. The liver infection was so painful that it made driving impossible and compelled him to travel for long periods prostrate on the back seat of a car. Nothing, however, was going to stop him from giving a talk at the Black Lion Hospital in Addis Ababa, Ethiopia. Godal may have looked pale after his arduous journey, and when he approached the lectern, he held up a urine container and said to the audience, 'this is not Coca-Cola, this is my urine, so if I faint during the lecture, you'll know why'.[48] Godal's prodigious career would extend over five decades and began with his pioneering work on leprosy in Ethiopia in 1970. In relation to his commitment to global health, he once joked, 'I travelled far, because of my deep interest in tropical medicine. My interest became a chronic infection'.[49] Godal retained a lifelong attachment to Ethiopia; and the people he met, worked with, and treated there, remained in the forefront of his mind.

One of Godal's former colleagues from that period was the US infectious diseases physician Ken Brown, who in the early 1970s was running a government hospital, in Metu, a town in south-western Ethiopia. Brown was part of the US Presbyterian Mission Agency's health programme in Africa before taking a position at Merck Research Laboratories in the 1980s, where one of his roles was to write the first protocol for the human use of ivermectin. During the intervening years, the men had remained friends, and they now found themselves reunited in a common cause, discussing which organisation should be the custodian of the ivermectin donation programme. 'Tore is a remarkably agile person intellectually', Ken Brown recalls,

> and in all of the time I knew Tore, I never saw him get angry with anybody, or saw him treat anyone with disrespect. . . . With the ivermectin story, I became a reluctant intermediary between Roy (Vagelos) and Tore in a way that seemed quite strange to me. I do not even recall what the specific issue was that they needed to talk to each other about. But what would happen, Tore would say. 'I need to talk to Roy, what I should say?' Well, I would make some suggestions and he would write to Roy'. Then Roy would say to me, 'Ken I just got this note from Tore, what should I say?' I was in the strange position because Roy was somewhat cryptic.[50]

Fortunately, Ken Brown's actions as an interlocutor led to a consensus of thinking, and after the disinterest shown by both USAID and WHO, and on Godal's recommendation, Roy Vagelos approached the epidemiologist Bill Foege, head of the Task Force for Child Survival, to see if he would be take up the challenge of distributing ivermectin. Foege, who had seen the devastation caused by river blindness while living in rural Nigeria, willingly accepted the challenge on the condition that the programme would be overseen from his offices in Atlanta (Georgia, USA). The bequest was named the Mectizan Donation Programme (MDP). The initiative's design had a two-pronged approach: one termed 'the humanitarian donation', aimed at physicians who had patients they could treat individually, and the other, a less well-defined 'mass treatment' regime. In effect, Merck had launched the largest philanthropic drug donation venture in human history and at the same time created a separate NGO to manage the donation.[51] Part of the impact of the Mectizan Donation Programme has been to find new ways of marshalling the forces of the world to improve health. Bill Foege, in his concise and beautifully constructed book *The Task Force for Child Survival*, described how a coalition synthesised between the Task Force, the Mectizan Expert Committee, The World Bank and voluntary organisations formed a truly unique structure. 'It is one of the most unusual coalitions in the history of global health because it doesn't answer to the WHO, UNICEF, or other UN agencies'.[52] Foege was, and is, a towering figure in global health in every sense, having devised the ring vaccination strategy, to contain the spread of smallpox that led to the eradication of the disease in the 1970s. Bill Foege is one of Tore Godal's global health 'heroes', and both men wanted to find new ways of aligning the forces of the world to improve human health.

How Vision Led the Way

Throughout the second half of the twentieth century, assiduous work was being undertaken in Africa by charities and institutions dedicated to blindness rehabilitation. Blindness caused by onchocerciasis is irreversible, and it was common to see blind adults being led with a stick by their children. During this colonial period, while trade certainly followed the flag, so too did acts of philanthropy. In 1950, Sir John Wilson, a blind activist, founded the British Empire Society for the Blind – today better known as Sightsavers – and on a visit to Ghana, Wilson and his wife, Jean decided that they would raise money and draw attention to the plight of those affected by the shattering disease.[53] When I visited Lady Jean Wilson at her home, high on a bluff overlooking Brighton Marina, in the United Kingdom, the 95-year-old activist described with limpid clarity her indelible contribution to the classification of the disease.

> We were in Nakong, and the men were wandering around led by very thin children, and the women were using a hemp rope to guide themselves to the village well. The people thought that the blindness was to do with the flies and the main thing was the itching. . . . One day we were out, and our car got stuck in a riverbed. It was boiling hot, but the windows were kept shut to stop the flies from getting in. And John said, 'when we get back to England, we must do some research on this, I think it might be something called onchocerciasis. And I replied, *Onchocerciasis! I can't say it. I can't spell it. And I certainly couldn't raise funds for it.* And looking at all of the flies pinging on the river, I said 'John, could we call it river blindness? And the name sort of took off'.[54]

At the same time as Sightsavers was expanding its operations within the blind community, CBM (Christoffel-Blindenmission) and the International Eye Foundation were also conducting valuable work focused on preventing and curing blindness at the community level. This practical hands-on experience became the platform upon which the new disease control programme was built.

Arguably, the mantra most associated with the disease is 'river blindness begins where the road ends', and it was in these distant locations that community ophthalmologists brought eye care services, cataract surgery and other prevention of blindness activities. This was to prove invaluable, as several the individuals whose experience was gained in the pre-ivermectin era, made a permanent contribution to the philosophy, design and intellectual currency of the African Programme for Onchocerciasis Control (APOC). Coming from the *vision* side, rather than the *disease* side of river blindness, they were well versed in the sensibilities of the communities which they served. These trusted ophthalmologists, who included among others Bjorn Thylefors, Adrian Hopkins, Yankum Dadzie and Allen Foster, had been working in blindness prevention programmes since the 1970s, and would go on to become highly influential within the hierarchy of river blindness control programmes.

The African Programme for Onchocerciasis Control (APOC)

In 1974, Bjorn Thylefors was a founding member of OCP living in Ouagadougou. His job was to travel around with parasitologists to map the disease and establish control villages for parasitological assessment and detailed ophthalmic evaluations. Six years later, he joined the Programme for Blindness Prevention at the WHO and became its manager in 1981. For the next 20 years, he used his position to encourage the use of ivermectin, to build the infrastructure for its distribution with NGOs and to forge relationships with Ministries of Health in the 31 onchocerciasis-endemic countries in Africa and across the globe. From the outset, for Thylefors, organisation was the key, and he built up a good working relationship with the NGOs that would be essential to the success of his programme.

> They had the advantage that they worked at the community level, and they knew what they were talking about in terms of practical experience. That is not something that you can learn in books. The NGOs did very well, they came in and they developed much of this practical approach in the villages.[55]

At the same time as Thylefors was coordinating strategies in Geneva, Adrian Hopkins, a member of CBM, was working with river blindness patients in isolated villages in the north-west of the Central African Republic. His aim was to establish a national programme for Blindness Prevention, but the emergent availability of ivermectin was beginning to change treatment possibilities for NGOs; no longer was it a simple question of blindness rehabilitation, but what could be done to prevent blindness in the first place. The reality of this transformation in treatment presented itself in a life-changing moment for Hopkins when he visited an isolated community on a riverbank at the end of a road:

> I walked from the vehicle and asked 'is anyone in the village blind?' I saw 34 blind people that afternoon and I couldn't do anything for them. That was the turning point for me. Suddenly I realised how important this disease was: in some of these villages, 50% of adults were blind, and obviously, this led to a downward economic spiral. Young people started leaving, as they did not want to live in these circumstances. Although I had seen the disease before, I had never seen that impact on a whole community before. That was what pushed me to make a major effort to get ivermectin to people – that is what got me into it.[56]

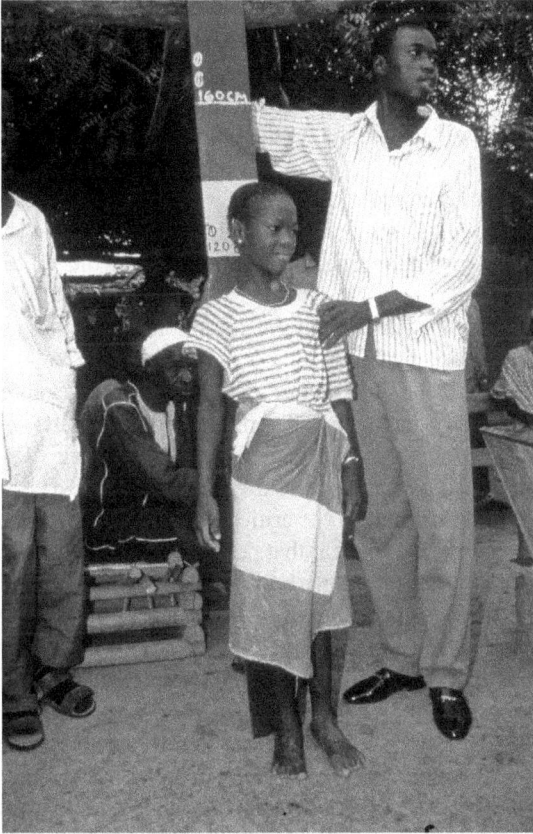

Figure 2.3 A young girl being measured with a Dose Pole in Mali, in 1996. This was at a time when 6 mg ivermectin tablets were being used – hence, the 2-tablet image on the pole for people over 160 cm. Merck later supplied ivermectin in 3 mg tablets which made it easier to give appropriate dose ranges.

Source: Courtesy of Andy Crump.

OCP introduced the distribution of ivermectin in regions where the programme operated, while at the same time governments and non-governmental development organisations (NGDOs) began distribution programmes in highly endemic areas beyond the remit of OCP in Central and East Africa.[57] There were some predictable problems in the early days of the drug's use. For example, the first tablets delivered by Merck were in six-milligram measurements: too high a dose. Workers in the field had to divide the tablets in half before they could be given to patients. However, within 12 months, this problem had been remedied, and the company delivered the required three-milligram tablets in boxes of 100 or 500 treatments, which was a great improvement. This modification was in response to some innovative research into the dose schedule of ivermectin.[58] The drug was given on a weight-adjusted basis, which meant that every patient had to be weighed before treatment. This was a difficult task when working in remote locations, so the researchers carried out a study-defining dose by height in Nigeria, Malawi and Guatemala. As the report stated,

> height can be measured more easily than weight; in fact, it can be done with a piece of string with knots or a stick with notches at 95 and 125cm. A 3mg tablet would also give appropriate dose ranges and avoid splitting tablets.

The findings led to the introduction of the ubiquitous dose poles as a simple way to determine drug dosage by height.

Judicious post-treatment surveillance was carried out to ensure that the drug was safe and free of any damaging side effects. This came at a time when there had been reports that some people had fainted after taking ivermectin. These patients could conceivably have been suffering from other diseases in addition to onchocerciasis, but it remained of critical importance to evaluate the drug's efficacy across populations. The fear that people might faint and hurt themselves was removed by the practical advice of the Director of OCP, Ebrahim Samba, when he promoted the idea that 'Mectizan day is a day of rest'. The idea was that after treatment, the patient was expected not to return to work, but to rest.[59] Dr Samba was an extremely effective and highly respected figure in global health politics, who, according to Tore Godal, 'had the people's trust'.[60] Bill Campbell looked upon Ebrahim Samba as an 'absolutely terrific' figure, who played a vital role in the dialogue with Roy Vagelos leading up to the donation of the drug. Indeed, if ivermectin's miraculous efficacy enabled it to transcend national borders, Ebrahim Samba's dedication to the health of Africa was so respected that his influence within the continent seemed almost unbounded. On one of his many journeys into the field, Bill Campbell witnessed the nexus of goodwill that Dr Samba had engendered for the control of the disease, even in the most combustible of political circumstances: '[even]when countries were at war, Ebrahim Samba enabled "*Oncho*" [marked] cars to cross borders. I crossed in one of these cars: if you were "*Oncho*", you were alright'.[61]

Ivermectin is an extremely safe broad-spectrum drug, and with over 30 million infected people spread throughout Africa, workers in the field began to question whether they really needed to make a diagnosis in each case before treatment. The adoption of this policy would mean the rejection of the traditional role of the physician, who expected to examine a patient, diagnose the illness and treat it accordingly. What is more, many of the founding designers of APOC had been trained in public health, and were prepared to advocate a community, public health dimension for the treatment of the disease. The recognition that Mectizan was much safer than aspirin removed another worry for those working in the field. Except for areas where Loa loa, another filarial disease, was also

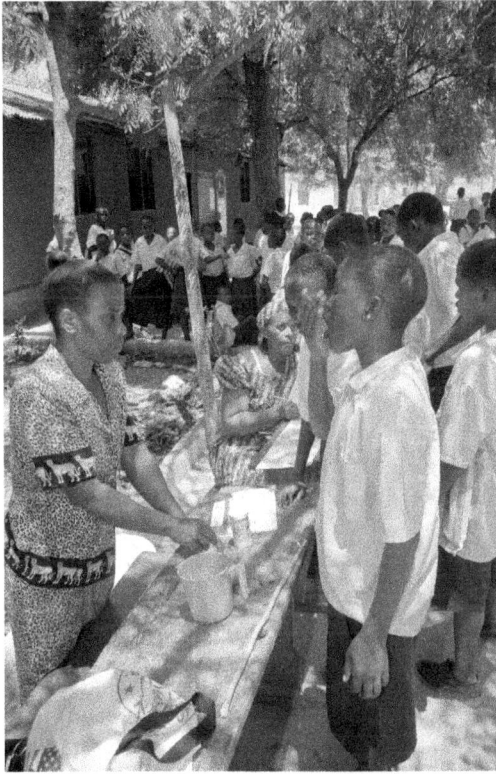

Figure 2.4 Tanzanian schoolchildren taking part in the first nationwide administration of ivermectin for the treatment of onchocerciasis, plus albendazole to combat lymphatic filariasis, commonly known as elephantiasis, in 2006.

Source: Courtesy of Andy Crump.

present, it was perfectly safe to give the drug. More crucially, the health gain for infected children multiplied, as ivermectin was also effective against lymphatic filariasis and scabies, resulting in improved intellectual acuity, increased school attendance and performance. 'Because of that', as Adrian Hopkins observes, 'you don't have to be quite so concerned with the question of whether you are treating someone who doesn't need treatment'.[62]

APOC was one of the rare programmes – the other being polio – that the WHO implemented directly, through the Regional Office for Africa (AFRO) and the APOC Secretariat located in Ouagadougou, Burkina Faso.[63] The African Programme for Onchocerciasis Control's formation came as a direct result of the donation of ivermectin and predicated on the idea that by controlling the disease this would eliminate the suffering and poverty it caused. Critical to the success of the programme was the efficient distribution of ivermectin, with the long-term goal of building a reliable structure of distribution that might eventually be utilised to treat other tropical diseases. This method of treatment, known as Mass Drug Administration (MDA), is active today, and had been advocated as early as 1990 by the tropical diseases physician, Kenneth Warren, for the control of the major human helminth parasites.[64] APOC's creation represented a new strategic template for public health; a prodigious social and medical experiment planned by an idealistic generation steeped in the spirit of public service. In 1992, some of these individuals formed the Non-Governmental Development Organizations (NGDOs) Coordinating Group for Ivermectin Distribution to improve coordination among themselves.[65] At the epicentre of this administrative creation was the Ghanaian ophthalmologist Yankum Dadzie, who after spending the previous 12 years working in Ouagadougou was ideally suited to the role of harmonising the move of NGDOs into Thylefors' Prevention of Blindness Unit in Geneva. The NGDO group was chaired by Allen Foster and included among others Sightsavers, CBM and The International Eye Foundation. This new partnership, comprising like-minded, forward-thinking individuals, was an ideal cohort for the equally principled Yankum Dadzie to join:

> I transferred to Geneva, and was coordinating the activities in the countries outside OCP where ivermectin was being used to control onchocerciasis. My relationship with the NGDOs in Geneva was very friendly and with Allen Foster, Bjorn, Bruce Benton from the World Bank, and advice from Brian Duke, we discussed the concept of creating a new OCP, and that's how APOC was formed.[66]

In December 1995, the World Bank launched the African Programme for Onchocerciasis Control (APOC) and acted as its fiscal agent. A key financial instrument for managing APOC's finances was its Trust Fund, a mechanism by which seven donors co-financed international development projects.

Community-Directed Treatment With Ivermectin (CDTI)

If, as Bill Campbell believes, 'it really is an arm's race' between humanity and disease, then APOC's strategic defence initiative was the community-based approach.[67] This had become possible through the large randomized community-based trials carried out by TDR that showed that ivermectin was very safe and therefore could be distributed by volunteers. Community-Directed Treatment with Ivermectin (CDTI) was a TDR innovation founded on sound epidemiological studies of treatment given by volunteers across several African countries.[68] At a stroke, this system removed the need to have an expensively trained physician supervise the distribution of the drug, and by scaling up drug delivery through community participation, it solved the infrastructure problem, making mass drug administration (MDA) possible. By devolving power to the community, APOC was built on the idea of sustainability; collectively its leadership recognised that those who truly wanted to end the cycle of infection, blindness and penury were the communities most at risk of contracting the disease.[69]

The scientific foundations of CDTI came from the work of the Dutch mathematician and epidemiologist Hans Remme. He brought the APOC-participating countries together and encouraged them to come up with ideas that he could test in the field. From the outset, two parallel drug delivery systems were in operation, one very regimented in design, involving centrally trained national coordinators who were transported to the villages. Their modus operandi was to assemble all of the villagers, treat them and then move on to the next village. Conversely, the NGDOs as witnessed by Yankum Dadzie, did things differently.

They trained one person, put them in the village and slowly that one person convinced people how the treatment worked, and how it would benefit the community. And that one person managed to treat more people than the regimental method. The idea then developed that if we could make the villagers themselves think 'this drug is available, this is something we can do for ourselves, and this is how we want to do it' then it would probably be a good thing.[70]

Following this discovery, Remme together with a team of social scientists designed a study across eight countries lasting three years; the experiment was divided into two evaluating wings, a top-down approach as opposed to asking villagers to coordinate drug distribution.[71] After three years, the evidence was compelling: 'it became very clear from the analysis that when the villagers accepted and understood what to do, the coverage was much better and their sustainability too was much higher'.[72] Earlier in the century, the medical missionary John G. Grant had pioneered the training of barefoot doctors in China, and now in Africa a new group of dedicated individuals were selected to serve the needs of their communities. This volunteer army of community-directed distributors was an educative force, calling door-to-door, distributing annual treatments of ivermectin throughout the 19 countries that comprised APOC. The main criteria with which these essential Community Drug Distributors were selected were 'trust, honesty, and reliability'.[73] The community-directed response was the human dynamic powering APOC forward, giving it, unlike OCP, a completely self-perpetuating local African identity. Strengthening the role of Africans in their own health care was pivotal to APOC's success according to the medical entomologist Daniel Boakye.

The idea that you could let community members take charge of their own treatment was revolutionary – it was a rejection of conventional medical training, and overcame the problem of treating people in very remote places where there were no medical facilities. The community directed programme was the icing on the cake, allowing coverage in all the nooks and crannies of Africa, and making it possible to scale-up the treatment.[74]

The unique design structure and effectiveness of APOC led to it being described as, 'one of the most successful public-private partnerships for health in Africa'.[75]

Perhaps more than any other individual, the Nigerian social scientist Uche Amazigo was responsible for emphasizing skin disease as an important part of river blindness. While a PhD student supported by TDR, Uche Amazigo visited clinics looking for river blindness patients. She observed they were itching a lot. 'It was like Newton seeing the implications of the apple falling', observed Godal 'suddenly the skin manifestations became the centre of attention because just like leprosy with its skin manifestations it had such severe social consequences with stigmatization and exclusion'.[76] Amazigo subsequently also became the champion of the idea of empowering communities into becoming the backbone of onchocerciasis control in Africa.[77] 'Community ownership' was what Amazigo had in mind as the mechanism for empowering Africans to formally play a part in their own health care.[78] River blindness is a dermatological disease before it is an eye disease, and Amazigo's study on the social influence of disfigurement among adolescent girls added a new dimension to the understanding of the impact of the infection.[79] For Amazigo, the only woman to have been Director of APOC (2005–2011), this work on the stigma of skin disease in village communities was to be a formative experience.

> I had learned a lot from community women about how skin disease affected their lives, and from then on I realised that listening to the poor would give us a very useful insight into solutions to their problems and how to engage them to be part of that solution.[80]

Amazigo was resistant to the idea of externally driven treatment programmes, involving well-dressed field workers in ostentatious vehicles making intermittent visits to communities and thereby destroying the spirit of participation that she believed would be Africa's salvation. As a careful and practical scientist, she quickly recognised the potential of community mobilisation. If correctly implemented,

> mobilisation does not mean one visit to the community. It means patiently repeating the visits, engaging people, training them, and allowing the community to appoint and select the community distributors. When you invest in community building, getting the communities to hold their own meetings, you then get people involved who become not just recipients but active participants in finding solutions. In the early days of APOC we had a good understanding of the values of community, good mobilisation and sensitisation. We made a deliberate effort to increase the workforce of women as ivermectin distributors even in areas where women were in purdah; we tried our best to find strategies to engage them.[81]

A symbiosis existed between Uche Amazigo's studies and the social and economic research (SER) championed by Godal at TDR. Hans Remme, together with Carol

Vlassoff and Mitchell Weiss, produced influential studies on community-directed treatment of ivermectin, the emerging field of cultural epidemiology, and on gender and stigma of onchocercal skin disease in Africa.[82] Of course, the real heroes of the APOC story were these community workers distributing the drug year-on-year. In recompense, the community might reward these workers with crops, or the use of a bicycle, or occasionally a small amount of money. However, the true value of their dedication was the respect and acclaim in which their community held them.[83]

Mapping and Treatment

The communities with the highest risk of contracting the disease desperately needed ivermectin. Identifying these communities was helped immensely by the application of the rapid epidemiological mapping of onchocerciasis (REMO).[84] Essentially this method analysed two variables; the proximity of communities to blackfly breeding sites and surveys carried out in sampled villages using a rapid assessment method based on the prevalence of nodules on the body to assess whether the area was hyper endemic. The nodules, due to the presence of the adult worms, which usually appear on the head, are in fact small nests where the worms twist themselves up together into balls. This system of mapping had the advantage of avoiding the more accurate but time consuming and very painful system of prevalence mapping: taking a skin snip and counting the number of microfilaria under a microscope. Using this 'community diagnosis' strategy, nodule counts in villages were used to decide the trigger points at which treatment would begin: usually at around a figure of 20%.[85] CDTI was formally adopted by APOC in 1997 as its principal strategy. The scaling up of this policy was spearheaded by the NGDOs, who had contributed so significantly to the development of CDTI, and whose strength came from working together with communities and governments in endemic countries.

Achievement and Legacy 1995–2015

Within a decade of its launch, APOC had successfully expanded coverage to a population of over 100 million people and treated 80% of the populations at risk.[86] By the time the programme closed at the end of 2015, it had trained more than 148,000 health workers, 1.46 million community-directed distributors, and delivered more than one billion treatments across the continent.[87] Only 42 years after Robert McNamara's visit to Burkina Faso, APOC's singular achievement is that, with the possible exception of South Sudan, onchocerciasis is no longer a blinding disease in Africa.[88] As a public health strategy, it could not be simpler, to deliver one dose, once a year to 100 million people.[89] APOC was also an outstanding example of a successful African health programme. As an entity, it was entirely embedded in the continent of Africa: an African owned, managed and run organisation where donors went to Africa for meetings. It was chaired by the Regional Director of WHO and had the participation of African Ministers of

Health. At the same time, APOC's existence was due to substantial engagement and support from the global north in the form of partnerships of various sorts, encompassing NGDO's, academic institutions and a World Bank Trust Fund.

Poverty is still the single biggest obstacle to improving health in the developing world, and in Africa some populations remain too poor to distribute free drugs. As running a successful Mass Drug Distribution Programme requires, among other things, scientific support, a communications network and logistics to transport medicines from central stores to outlying villages, a lack of capacity in terms of human and financial resources affects many regions.[90] This reality should not detract from the lasting influence of APOC on strategies to control NTDs, and the impact of ivermectin on infectious diseases. The Australian pathologist Charles Mackenzie worked on onchocerciasis in Ecuador and Sudan in the days before ivermectin, when treatment with diethylcarbamazine (DEC) could be fatal[91] and has no doubt about the transformative power of the drug. 'The big thing about ivermectin . . . was that it changed the world'.[92] The drug's discovery led inexorably to Merck's donation, which was initially envisaged to reach 45 million treatments annually but escalated to over 100 million per year. This was a decisive event in combating what had been described in 1977 as 'the great neglected diseases of mankind'.[93] The effect was transformative; the burden of disease began to diminish, with some indigenous parasitic diseases becoming for the first time a thing of the past. This reality was a vindication of the contribution made by public and private partnerships, non-governmental development organisations and by the donation of ivermectin which made APOC possible. Simon Bush, Sightsavers' Accra-based Director of NTDs has observed at first hand the revolutionary impact of the programme:

> One of the most powerful messages that I got was in northern Ghana, where I regularly meet with community leaders to talk about these diseases and what the communities are doing. I was talking about one disease, and the community said 'we haven't got that anymore' – now that was far more important to me than reading some piece of research or some surveillance that actually said 'the community in the Yendi district hasn't got river blindness anymore'.[94]

Moreover, the successful control of onchocerciasis inspired a bigger vision for NTDs, one that, while owing much to APOC's accomplishments, would eventually supersede the programme and make it redundant. By the beginning of the twenty-first century, a new ethos in tackling the challenges of developing world disease was discernible in global health thinking. The psychology of pharmaceutical companies had been altered by APOC's success and by Merck's donation programme, with others now also keen to contribute. The tipping point came when SmithKlineBeecham (later GlaxoSmithKline (GSK)) entered the field. In 1997, the WHO Assembly passed a resolution calling for the global elimination of lymphatic filariasis (LF) (also known as elephantiasis). In the same year, SmithKlineBeecham formed a pioneering collaboration with WHO that had one

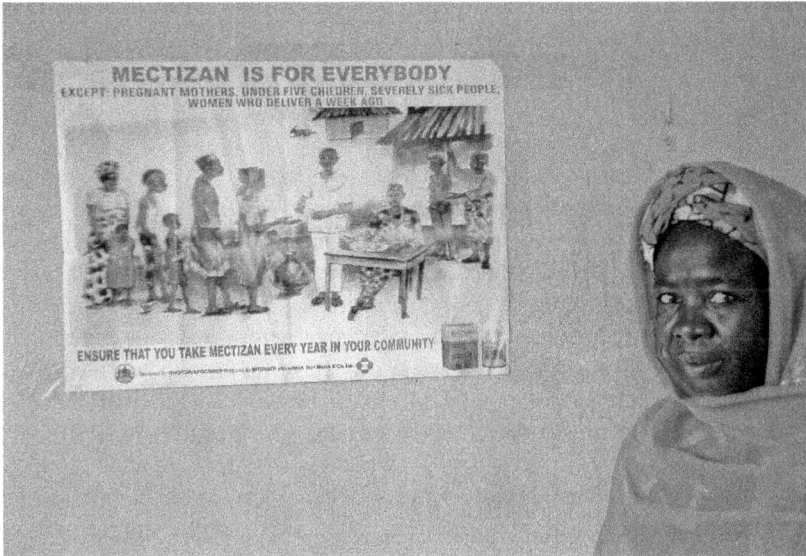

Figure 2.5 A nutrition teacher in Nigeria stands beside a public information poster before giving a talk to local villagers in 2007.

Source: Courtesy of Andy Crump.

simple goal – to eliminate LF as a public health problem via the donation of Albendazole. In 2000, the newly formed GSK joined the WHO as a founder member of the LF Global Alliance, a public–private partnership which saw Merck providing Mectizan to the countries in Sub-Saharan Africa where LF and river blindness co-existed. Thus, in the arena of NTDs, a landmark transformation was taking place; former competitors were becoming partners, and soon others would follow, eager to become active participants in a common cause. In 1998, Pfizer, makers of the antibiotic Zithromax, and the Edna McConnell Clark Foundation, under the leadership of Joe Cook, co-established the International Trachoma Initiative (ITI), dedicated to eliminating trachoma by 2020. Trachoma and LF are more widespread diseases than onchocerciasis, affecting more people in larger geographies, and their inclusion in donation programmes elevated NTDs still further in global health politics and at the WHO. In September 2005, Lorenzo Savioli was appointed Director of the newly constituted Department of Neglected Tropical Diseases of WHO, an obvious marker of the growing status of NTDs on the global health agenda.

During his tenure as director of the Mectizan Donation Programme (2001–2007), Bjorn Thylefors established the influential Partnership for Disease Control Initiatives, composed of representatives of the medical donor programmes and a venue where the MDP, GSK, Pfizer, Johnson & Johnson, Sanofi Aventis and other companies could meet twice a year for small informal discussions. It is still in existence today and has grown considerably in size over the past decade as more pharmaceutical companies have entered the NTD field. For Bjorn Thylefors, the amenable atmosphere of these meetings enhanced the spirit of collaboration that was a growing feature among the donor companies.

> The meetings were small, about fifteen or twenty people, and it gave us time and the opportunity to talk about all of the things between us, the common experiences and issues such as customs registration, import controls and batch number verifications. It gave you an opportunity to realise that you were not alone as a donor programme and that you could perhaps gain something from working with the other person across the table. It did wonders for the relationship between GSK and Merck for example, as it was much better for them to transport Mectizan and Albendazole more or less jointly into the countries. There was an interest in trying to collaborate instead of everybody doing their own business.[95]

Translating discoveries made in the laboratory into drugs to treat people who are sick remains a high priority for Tore Godal and other global health researchers. 'One view', Godal has written 'that I heard then [the 1980s] as well as repeatedly throughout my career was: "We have the tools we need, it is only a question of application"'.[96] However, this was not the case, and Godal's work showed unambiguously that research, and discovery science played a decisive role in bringing innovations in health. In addition, the economist and global health strategist, Dean Jamison, believes that Tore Godal's leadership of TDR 'seemed a model for helping WHO shed its aversion to dealing with the private sector'.[97] Of course, much still needs to be done, as more than one billion people are affected by neglected tropical diseases worldwide, diminishing productive capacity and trapping communities in cycles of poverty.

From APOC to the London Declaration

The APOC programme was originally envisaged to end in 2010, but just as its predecessor, the OCP, had been given an operational extension, APOC did not end its community-directed treatment with ivermectin until 2015. The programme was successful in treating at least 80% of targeted populations, but received criticism for not persuading African governments to provide more support to sustain disease treatments[98] and for other serious shortcomings. APOC's sister programme, the Onchocerciasis Elimination Programme for the Americas (OEPA), started in 1992, has verified four countries (Guatemala, Ecuador, Mexico and Columbia) free of transmission of river blindness. This feat, achieved admittedly in smaller geographies with far less disease endemicity, was not realised by APOC, and while elimination became an objective of APOC in 2009, it had no tangible evidence to show partners that elimination of transmission had been accomplished in any one specific country. The second major problem undermining APOC was that during the 20 years of the programme's existence, the economic, pharmaceutical and philanthropic landscape had changed. While APOC had been a success, its *modus operandi* was gradually undermined by the emergence of a new popular mood within strategic health care thinking which advocated a move towards an integrated NTD programme.

At the same time as APOC began the process of winding down its operations, in January 2012, an exclusive gathering in London, 'Uniting to Combat Neglected Tropical Diseases', announced a new public–private partnership to eliminate or control preventable NTDs.[99] The meeting led to the 'London Declaration on NTDs', which marked a turning point in the history of neglected diseases. The meeting, co-chaired by Bill Gates, from the Bill and Melinda Gates Foundation, and Sir Andrew Witty, CEO of GlaxoSmithKline, brought together 13 pharmaceutical companies to enhance private-sector investment in public health challenges. The decision was taken by the world's largest pharmaceutical companies, including Merck in conjunction with the WHO, to eliminate or control the ten most common NTDs. This unprecedented donation programme was an affirmation to end the suffering and impoverishment caused by Guinea worm, LF, leprosy, sleeping sickness (human African trypanosomiasis) blinding trachoma, river blindness, soil transmitted helminths, schistosomiasis, visceral leishmaniasis and Chagas disease.[100] Five of the ten diseases were to be addressed via preventive chemotherapy (PC-NTDs), the system pioneered by APOC.

This was the background to the evolution of a new integrated programme for the elimination of NTDs in Africa. New ideas needed a new acronym, and in May 2016, ESPEN (the Expanded Special Project for Elimination of Neglected Tropical Diseases) was launched as a new partnership with NGDOs and the pharmaceutical industry, with a defining emphasis on country ownership of health infrastructure, including decision-making and financing.[101] ESPEN thus provided an answer to earlier criticisms that APOC depended too much on funding from international agencies.[102] The example of the Mectizan® donation programme stimulated large-scale drug donation programmes from additional pharmaceutical companies for the treatment of other neglected tropical diseases, and was a forerunner of the Global Fund to Fight AIDS, Tuberculosis and Malaria. Reflecting a recognition that countries afflicted by the diseases of poverty would need innovative mechanisms to provide treatments that by themselves, they would be unable to afford.

The contemporary history of attempts to control and eliminate river blindness has many pertinent lessons for us today as we continue to develop strategies to eliminate NTDs across the globe. It would serve us well to recognise the lasting contribution made by those working in the field before the discovery of ivermectin, who subsequently used their expertise, intellectual capital and idealism to chart a course for the control and possible elimination not only of onchocerciasis but for other NTDs in Africa and beyond. Meanwhile, the discovery and donation of ivermectin reminds us not simply of the transformative power of well-funded medical research but also that this force can often be most effectively harnessed and deployed in an alliance with the philanthropic ideal. The leadership shown by Merck & Company (Rahway, NJ) to donate the drug for as long as it was needed was the catalyst for other pharmaceutical companies to follow in Merck's tradition. A decisive element in this research, led by TDR, was overcoming the problem of how to distribute ivermectin at scale within rural communities. As a result, community-directed treatment was born, and its legacy firmly established in global health policy. Finally, the shift in attitudes, towards community-based medicine, and then on a broader scale in favour of African countries developing their own elimination programmes and health infrastructure, acts as an indicator of the huge potential for the developed and developing world to work in equal and mutual partnership.

Notes

1. D. A. P. Bundy, "How will the Nobel scientists transform medicine?", *The Agenda Weekly, World Economic Forum*, 2015, pp. 1–6.
2. H. Ridley, *British Journal of Ophthalmology*, 1945, 29 (Suppl), pp. 3–38.
3. Interview with Adrian Hopkins, April 2016.
4. J. P. McMahon, R. B. Highton, H. H. Goiny, "The eradication of *Simulium neavei* from Kenya", *Bulletin of the World Health Organization*, 1958, 18, pp. 75–107.
5. J. Hissett, "Sur l'existence d'affections oculaires importantes d'origine filarienne dans certains territoires du Congo", *Annales de la Societe Belg de Medicine Tropicale*, 1931, 11, pp. 45–46.
6. H. Ridley, "Ocular onchocerciasis, including an investigation in the Gold Coast", *British Journal of Ophthalmology*, Monograph supplement, 1945, 10, p. 58.
7. J. P. McMahon, R. B. Highton, H. H. Goiny, "The eradication of *Simulium neavei* from Kenya", *Bulletin of the World Health Organization*, 1958, 18, pp. 75–107.
8. J. B. Davies, "Sixty years of onchocerciasis vector control: A chronological summary with comments on eradication, reinvasion, and insecticide resistance", *Annual Review of Entomology*, 1994, 39, pp. 23–45.
9. *The British Simuliid Group Bulletin*, No. 36 July 2011, 5.
10. Interview with Bjorn Thylefors, May 2016.
11. Interview with Allen Foster, April 2016.
12. Interview with John Davis, June 2016.
13. D. A. P. Bundy, B. Dhomun, X. Daney, L. B. Shultz, A. Tembon, "Investing in onchocerciasis control: Financial management of the African Programme for Onchocerciasis Control (APOC)", *Public Library of Science Neglected Tropical Diseases*, 2015, 9 (5), p. e0003508.
14. Interview with Azodoga Seketeli, July 2016.
15. H. Ridley, "Ocular onchocerciasis, including an investigation in the Gold Coast", *British Journal of Ophthalmology*, Monograph supplement, 1945, 10, p. 58.
16. K. Collins, "Profitable gifts: A history of the Merck Mectizan donation program and its implications for international health", *Perspectives in Biology and Medicine*, 2004, 47 (1), pp. 100–109.
17. G. W. Esch, *Parasites and Infectious Disease: Discovery by Serendipity, and Otherwise* (Cambridge: Cambridge University Press, 2007), 18.
18. The Nobel Prize in Physiology and Medicine in 2015 was shared between William Campbell and Satoshi Omura, and the Chinese researcher Tu Youyou for the discovery of artemisinin, a highly effective anti-malarial drug now used to treat millions of people every year. As the Nobel committee said in announcing the award, 'the consequences in terms of improved human health and reduced suffering are immeasurable'.

19. Interview with Bill Campbell, May 2016.
20. Interview with Bill Campbell, May 2016.
21. J. Lofflin, "The miracle molecule: The story of a Japanese golf course, a fluke soil sample, and one of the most important drugs in veterinary history", *Veterinary Medicine*, A Century of Change, 2005, A supplement to Veterinary Medicine.
22. Interview with Bill Campbell, May 2016.
23. Interview with Bill Campbell, May 2016.
24. Interview with Bill Campbell, May 2016.
25. W. C. Campbell, *The Genesis of the Antiparasitic Drug Ivermectin* (Oxford: Oxford University Press, 1992), pp. 194–214.
26. K. Collins, "Profitable gifts: A history of the Merck Mectizan donation program and its implications for international health", *Perspectives in Biology and Medicine*, 2004, 47 (1), pp. 100–109.
27. Interview with Bill Campbell, May 2016.
28. A. O. Lucas, *It Was the Best of Times: From Local to Global Health* (Africa: Book-Builders, Editions, 2010), p. 246.
29. M. A. Aziz, S, Diallo, I. M. Diop, M. Lariviere, M. Porta, "Efficacy and tolerance of ivermectin in human onchocerciasis", *Lancet*, 1982, 2, p. 171.
30. Interview with Bill Campbell, May 2016.
31. Interview with Roy Vagelos, February 2016.
32. A. O. Lucas, *It Was the Best of Times: From Local to Global Health* (Africa: Book-Builders, Editions, 2010), p. 217.
33. Interview with Bjorn Thylefors, May 2016.
34. J. Goodfield *A Chance to Live: The Heroic Story of the Global Campaign to Immunize the World's Children* (New York: Macmillan, 1990), p. 3.
35. C. Keating, *Kenneth Warren and the Great Neglected Diseases of Mankind Programme: The Transformation of Geographical Medicine in the US and Beyond* (New York: Springer, 2017).
36. M. Cueto, "The Origins of Primary Health Care and Selective Primary Health Care", *American Journal of Public Health*, 2004, 44 (11), p. 3.
37. Primary Health Care, *A Joint Report by the Director-General of the World Health Organisation and the Executive Director of the United Nations Children's Fund* (New York: WHO, 1978).
38. Interview with Peter Smith, December 2019.
39. Interview with Tore Godal, March 2020.
40. Interview with Chris Murray, February 2019.
41. Tropical disease research: progress 1975–94, highlights 1993–94 twelfth programme report of the UNDP/World Bank/WHO Special Programme for Research and Training in Tropical Diseases (TDR). WHO (1995). 92.
42. Interview with Tore Godal, March 2020.
43. A. Crump, "Tore Godal: Pragmatic opportunist championing global public health", *Trends in Parasitology*, 2006, 22 (8), p. 379.
44. Tropical disease research: progress 1975–94, highlights 1993–94 twelfth programme report of the UNDP/World Bank/WHO Special Programme for Research and Training in Tropical Diseases (TDR). WHO (1995). 92.
45. M. R. Reich, T. Fujisaki, "Assessment of TDR's contributions to product development for tropical diseases: The case of ivermectin for onchocerciasis", Prepared for the UNDP/World Bank/WHO Special Programme for Research and Training in Tropical Diseases (TDR) for the Third External Review of the Programme Activities, 1997.
46. Interview with Tore Godal, November 2019.
47. Letter from Antony Cerami of The Rockefeller University to Tore Godal dated 2 August 1988.
48. Email communication, Tore Godal, May 2021.

49. Interview with Helga Fogstad, June 2020.
50. Interview with Kenneth Brown, May 2021.
51. Interview with Allen Foster, April 2016.
52. W. H. Foege, *The Task Force for Child Survival: Secrets of Successful Coalitions* (Baltimore, MD: Johns Hopkins University Press, 2018), p. 104.
53. John Wilson was blinded in a school chemistry accident at the age of 12. He downplayed his blindness referring to it as 'a confounded nuisance', and his blindness did not prevent him from leading a successful life. He learned Braille, and while at the University of Oxford he lived a full undergraduate life, rowing for his college, becoming a noted dancer, and chairing the poetry society. But while he was travelling in Africa after World War II, he witnessed how blind people were often summarily dismissed as being unproductive members of society. This made him angry and led to him to establish the charity *The British Empire Society for the Blind* to confront this social injustice.
54. Interview with Lady Jean Wilson. November 2017.
55. Interview with Bjorn Thylefors, May 2016.
56. Interview with Adrian Hopkins, April 2016.
57. Interview with Adrian Hopkins, April 2016.
58. H. R. Taylor, C. Ganzales, B. Duke, "Simplified dose schedule of ivermectin", *Lancet*, 1993, 341, pp. 50–51.
59. Interview with Bjorn Thylefors, April 2016.
60. Interview with Tore Godal, August 2020.
61. Interview with William Campbell, May 2016.
62. Interview with Adrian Hopkins, April 2016.
63. D. A. P. Bundy, B. Dhomun, X. Daney, L. B. Shultz, A. Tembon, "Investing in onchocerciasis control: Financial management of the African Programme for Onchocerciasis Control (APOC)", *Public Library of Science Neglected Tropical Diseases*, 2015, 9 (5), p. e0003508.
64. K. S. Warren, "An integrated system for the control of the major human helminth parasites", *Acta Leidensia*, 1990, 59 (1&2), pp. 433–442.
65. Assessment of TDR's Contributions to Product Development for Tropical Diseases: The Case of Ivermectin for Onchocerciasis. A Report Prepared by Tomoko Fujisaki and Michael R. Reich. Takemi Program in International Health, Harvard School of Public Health. February 12, 1997: 20.
66. Interview with Yankum Dadzie, July 2016.
67. Interview with William Campbell, May 2016.
68. WHO, Community Directed Treatment with Ivermectin – Report of a multi-country study. TDR Applied Field Research Reports. TDR/AFT/RP/**96**.1. 1996.
69. One of the medical dilemmas for the researchers was deciding which villages needed treatment. Bill Foege thought that the skin snip biopsy was too complex, and instead, for reasons of simplicity, advocated a system whereby men in villages would be asked to reveal their torso and if more than 20% of those examined presented with nodules then the village needed treatment. 'This', Foege said at the time, 'is good enough for now'.
70. Interview with Yankum Dadzie, July 2016.
71. WHO, Community Directed Treatment with Ivermectin – Report of a multi-country study. TDR Applied Field Research Reports. TDR/AFT/RP/96.1. 1996.
72. Interview with Yankum Dadzie, July 2016.
73. WHO, Community Directed Treatment with Ivermectin – Report of a multi-country study. TDR Applied Field Research Reports. TDR/AFT/RP/96.1. 1996.
74. Interview with Daniel Boakye, July 2016.
75. D. A. P. Bundy, B. Dhomun, X. Daney, L. B. Shultz, A. Tembon, "Investing in onchocerciasis control: Financial management of the African Programme for

Onchocerciasis Control (APOC)", *Public Library of Science Neglected Tropical Diseases*, 2015, 9 (5), p. e0003508.

76. Interview with Tore Godal, August 2018.
77. A. O. Lucas, *It Was the Best of Times: From Local to Global Health* (Ibadan: Book-Byukders, 2010), p. 341.
78. Interview with Uche Amazigo, July 2016.
79. U. Amazigo, "Onchoceriasis and women's reproductive health: indigenous and bio-medical concepts", *Tropical Doctor*, 1993, 23, pp. 149–151.
80. Interview with Uche Amazigo, July 2016.
81. Interview with Uche Amazigo, July 2016.
82. C. Vlassoff, M, Weiss, E. B. L. Ovuga, C. Eneanya, P. Titi Nwel, S. Sunday Babalola, A. K. Aweboba, B. Theophilus, P. Cofie, P. Shetabi, "Gender and the stigma of onchocercal skin disease in Africa", *Social Science and Medicine*, 2000, 50, pp. 1353–1368.
83. Interview with Azodoga Seketeli, July 2016.
84. J. H. F. Remme, "The African programme for onchocerciasis control: Preparing to launch", *Parasitology Today*, 1995, 1, p. 11.
85. Interview with Adrian Hopkins, May 2016.
86. A. Seketeli, G. Adcoye, A. Eyamba, E. Nnoruka, P. Drameh, U. V. Amazigo, M. Noma, F. Agboton, Y. Aholou, O. O. Kale, D. Y. Dadzie, "The achievements and challenges of the African Programme for Onchocerciasis Control (APOC)", *Annals of Tropical Medicine and Parasitology*, 2002, 96 (Suppl 1), pp. 15–28.
87. J. B. Roungou, L. Yameogo, C. Mwikisa, G. A. Boakye, D. A. P. Bundy, "40 years of the APOC partnership", *Public Library of Science Neglected Tropical Diseases*, 2015, 9, p. e0003562.
88. Interview with Simon Bush, May 2016.
89. Interview with Allen Foster, May 2016.
90. Interview with Andy Wright, June 2016.
91. A. P. Ooman, "Fatalities after treatment of onchocerciasis with diethlcarbamazine", *Transactions of The Royal Society of Tropical Medicine and Hygiene*, 1969, 63 (4), p. 548.
92. Interview with Charles Mackenzie, July 2017.
93. K. S. Warren, C. C. Jimenez (eds.), *The Great Neglected Diseases of Mankind Bio-medical Research Network: 1978–1988* (New York: The Rockefeller Foundation, 1998), p. 1.
94. Interview with Simon Bush, May 2016.
95. Bjorn Thylefors, personal communication.
96. T. Godal, "From AHRI to CEPI: On my journey in global health", A Publication for the 50th Anniversary Meeting of the Armauer Hansen Research Institute.
97. Interview with Dean Jamison, October 2020.
98. D. R. Hopkins, F. O. Richards, M. Katabarwa, "Whither onchocerciasis control in Africa?", *American Journal of Tropical Medicine and Hygiene*, 2005, 72 (1), pp. 1–2.
99. D. A. P, Bundy, B. Dhomun, X. Daney, L. B. Schultz, A. Tembon, "Investing in onchocerciasis control: Financial management of the African Programme for Onchocerciasis Control (APOC)", *Public Library of Science Neglected Tropical Diseases*, 9 (5), p. e0003508.
100. Allen Foster, personal communication.
101. Adrian Hopkins, personal communication.
102. D. R. Hopkins, F. O. Richards, M. Katabarwa, "Whither onchocerciasis control in Africa?", *American Journal of Medicine and Hygiene*, 2005, 72 (1), pp. 1–2.

3 The Fall and Rise of Malaria

Short-term economic benefits from malaria control can be up to $12 billion each year. These are staggering numbers and there is no doubt that malaria is taking a big bite out of Africa's economic growth.[1]

Jeffrey Sachs

In 1949, an international congress on malaria coincided with the publication of Mark F Boyd's massive two-volume work on the science of malariology. Placing the tomes on the rostrum, Paul F Russell announced to the delegates, 'I present you these volumes as tombstones on the grave of malaria'.[2] More than 70 years later, however, it is apparent that Russell's optimism was misplaced: malaria and the mosquitoes that carry this deadly parasitic disease still refuse to be buried. Nevertheless, malaria is a preventable disease, and following the World Health Organization's failed eradication attempts in the 1950s and 1960s, global mortality and morbidity have decreased substantially since the beginning of the new millennium. This transformation was brought about by the synthesis of ambitious programmes established by the wider malaria community that were aligned to the successful translation of biomedical science into far-reaching public health initiatives, principal among which are rapid diagnostic tests, artemisinin-based combination therapies and long-lasting insecticide-treated bed nets. Indeed, over the past 20 years malaria control has saved more than six million lives, with much of the reduction in mortality coming as a direct result of the widespread use of insecticide-treated bed nets (ITNs). But the profound life-saving importance of insecticide-treated bed nets was not a self-evident truth; their preventive value was only accepted as real, following a series of persuasive randomised controlled trials in the 1990s. As a consequence, these trials constitute decisive moments in global health because malaria was, and still is, the most devastating parasitic disease of humans, and its prevention is paramount.

DOI: 10.4324/9781003363859-4

Origins of the 1991 Cluster Randomised Trial

The insidious and widespread emergence of resistance to antimalarial drugs in the 1980s[3] led to renewed interest in the use of vector control measures. Bed nets are a very old method of reducing contacts between humans and vectors, and may have been used in the Middle East over 1,000 years ago,[4] but the modern application of long-lasting insecticide to fabrics as a means of personal protection against mosquito-borne diseases dates from World War II with the impregnation of bed nets and combat fatigues by the Soviet, German and US armies.[5]

Of all the parasitic diseases, malaria is the most dangerous, with its geographical spread falling disproportionately on the world's poorest inhabitants. Sub-Saharan Africa bears the greatest burden of cases and deaths, most of them in children younger than five years. This continuing and unacceptable human cost was the motivating factor that supercharged efforts to devise new methods to protect vulnerable populations, ranging from a scientifically sophisticated and highly expensive recombinant DNA vaccine[6] to the comparatively unrefined and low-tech insecticide-treated bed nets (ITNs). In some African countries, bed nets had been used as a protection against malaria in the expatriate population even though there was no evidence in the scientific literature that they worked.[7] In the 1980s, when the leading tropical disease scientist, Sir Brian Greenwood, arrived in The Gambia, West Africa, to become director of the UK Medical Research Council Laboratories, he was surprised by the ubiquity of bed net use compared to the situation in northern Nigeria where he had spent the previous 15 years.

> When I started working in the Farafenni area I was struck by how many villagers had a net, it emerged that there was, almost uniquely in Africa, a history of people using nets going back over several generations, as a means of personal protection against bites and lizards dropping on their heads, rather than for preventing malaria.[8]

Inspired by the social traditions of the local community, Greenwood and his colleagues began, a series of experiments, examining the mechanisms of action (repellency and killing) determining the dosage of different insecticides to access the potential of bed nets for disease control. Likewise, other studies in The Gambia,[9] Kenya, Guinea Bissau, the United Republic of Tanzania and Sierra Leone met the basic requirements for randomised controlled trials. In the years that followed, much of the research on the ability of ITNs to shield sleeping children from attack by feeding mosquitoes was undertaken in The Gambia, the smallest country in Africa.[10] Experiments with bed nets were also launched in other countries where malaria was a serious public health problem, including Mali and Papua New Guinea. Unfortunately, many of these investigations, primarily due to their small sample sizes, lacked statistical power and as a consequence the evidence of the protective ability of bed nets had come to be seen as contentious, while some field experiments were regarded as difficult to interpret and evaluate because of their scope, design and the use of different clinical and parasitological measurements.[11]

This was the scientific status quo that prefaced an informal meeting of the World Health Organization's *Division of Vector-Borne Diseases* on the use of impregnated bed nets, held in February 1989. Among the delegates attending the meeting in Geneva was Pedro Alonso, a physician and specialist in study design at the MRC's laboratory in The Gambia. 'Some of the trials that we looked at', Alonso, until recently the Director of the WHO Global Malaria Programme recalls,

> were the product of small numbers, and because of the play of chance, it was difficult to measure the magnitude of the effect between normal nets and insecticide-treated bed nets. . . . While other trials carried out by entomologists showed good impact on the number of mosquitoes, but were poor in picking up that there was a difference in disease [prevalence].[12]

One should remember that this was the very early days in the modern epidemiology of malaria research and the concept of randomised controlled trials was still novel.[13] Nonetheless, when the methodological shortcomings of some of the experiments were critically dissected by the epidemiologist, Louis Molineaux, an expert in malariometric indices in Africa, it had a chastening effect on the entomologist, Steven Lindsay, another member of the Gambian-based malaria research team. 'This great man', Lindsay relived in painful memory, 'ripped everything to pieces and we came away from that meeting with our heads bowed because although our studies were randomised and considered suitable, there was a lot of uncertainty in the air'.[14] Alonso too felt that the meeting marked a watershed in the evolution of their research;

> at that point the mood was clearly, actually bed nets don't do much, this meeting is not going to go anywhere, and that is when Chris Curtis said something that I will never forget. 'Of course five million Chinese people can't be wrong'. Because the Chinese were actually doing research into bed nets, but still, the conclusion of that WHO meeting was that bed nets will never become a public health tool for control of malaria in Africa.[15]

The official WHO report of the meeting ultimately gave a less pessimistic overview and referred to the use of insecticide-treated nets as an 'exciting possibility', but acknowledged that the scientific evidence of their effectiveness as a form of malaria control 'is still incomplete'.[16] To rectify this deficiency, a call was made for further studies to be carried out using treated nets under different disease transmission conditions and in combination with other measures. The report concluded that 'these trials should be carefully designed so that more solid scientific evidence can be produced on which to base and formulate modern control strategies'.[17] The forces that shape scientific research, be they material, political or technological, emerge over time and some represent breakthroughs while others, regarding global public health innovators, may be an illustration of the fascinating occurrence of having the right person in the right place at the right time. This was just such a case. When Pedro Alonso returned to The Gambia at the end of February 1989, he immediately set about designing an experiment that would provide reliable evidence on the effectiveness of mosquito nets. After weeks of careful planning, Alonso visited his boss, Brian Greenwood at the MRC laboratories in Fajara and outlined his plan to conduct a large study of insecticide-treated bed nets that would measure childhood mortality as an endpoint. Greenwood was very receptive to researchers who wanted to carry out useful research on the diseases of poor people that caused poverty, because that was the epidemiological field that had come to define his own career in global health. At the time, the three big killers of children in Africa were pneumonia, diarrhoeal disease and malaria and as the director of the MRC's laboratories, Greenwood's objective was to find practical cost-effective control measures

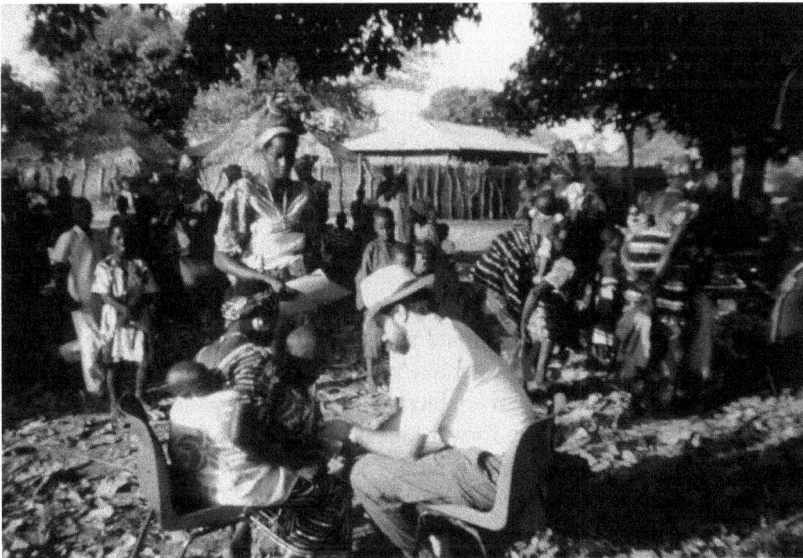

Figure 3.1 Malaria, the mosquito-borne disease, is a big killer of children particularly in Africa. In this photograph, taken in 1988, Pedro Alonso examines a child in one of the bed net villages on the north bank of the River Gambia.

Source: Courtesy of Alice Greenwood.

against these diseases. During the spring of 1989, Greenwood wrote a clear and uncomplicated trial protocol, and Alonso and Lindsay designed the methodology and management of the two-year project. The trialable hypothesis that the researchers designed their experiment to answer was clearly defined: were insecticide-treated bed nets an effective way of reducing mortality caused by malaria in Gambian children?

Intriguingly, while insecticide-treated bed nets offered the potential of being a cost-effective and simple method of reducing human contact with the mosquito vector, no previous study had shown their effect on mortality. The trial, which was to be led by Pedro Alonso, was going to be a large double intervention study of bed nets treated with the insecticide permethrin at the beginning of the malaria transmission season in villages taking part in a primary health care (PHC) scheme.[18] Additionally, children aged six months to five years were going to be randomised to receive seasonal malaria chemoprophylaxis with maloprim or a placebo throughout the transmission season. The idea was to measure the mortality in children in the PHC villages *before* and *after* the intervention. 'And the only really clever thing', according to Alonso who envisioned the study,

> although not randomised, we identified the villages that were geographically in between these PHC villages that would act as controls, so we would still have a comparison of ITNs bed nets plus nothing, versus just bed nets. But at the time we thought – no one would ever fund this trial!

Occasionally, luck favours daring experimenters, and four thousand kilometres north of The Gambia in an office in Geneva the trial's protocols were being studied with intellectual acuity by a global health public servant who would become the study's benefactor. Tore Godal, Director of the WHO Tropical Diseases Research Programme (known as TDR), immediately recognised the potential significance of the trial as a means of reducing childhood mortality. By creating a bridge between research, policy and operations, his objective was to save lives. When TDR was established in 1975, it had two key objectives: to develop new methods to prevent and treat tropical diseases, and to strengthen the capability of countries to undertake research related to the control of indigenous diseases.[19] Godal was an enabler, and under his stewardship TDR was a powerful organisation driving forward ideas in tropical research. As a result of the failure of the eradication programmes in the 1950s and 1960s, research in the field of malaria had stagnated; therefore, the arrival of an innovative and well-designed study immediately attracted Godal's attention. What appealed to him in particular was the ability to measure mortality as 'outcome' which is much more definite than measuring malaria cases which is particularly difficult in children is sub-Saharan Africa where over 90% of young children have parasites in their blood. Godal had taken up the leadership of TDR in 1986 and within a couple of years had become increasingly 'dismayed'[20] at WHO's ambiguous position on bed nets for malaria prevention. Having begun his career with pioneering research on leprosy in Ethiopia, Godal was dedicated to finding innovative ways to solve global health problems. Godal was conscious that one of his strategic roles was to promote investigations into the diseases of poverty or 'the parasites of poverty' as he notably referred to them, through public research.[21] He recognised that while it was the business of economics, politics and 'development' to deal with the root causes of tropical disease, he also believed that it was the business of health workers and concerned scientists to use all their means to alleviate the suffering caused by poverty and – the greatest challenge – to achieve effective results in the face of that poverty. Importantly for the researchers in The Gambia, Godal understood that one of the impediments to producing reliable scientific knowledge was the time and effort it took to raise sufficient funds to launch and manage a large study; therefore, using his powerful position of Director of TDR, Godal decided to underwrite the total cost of the two-year study. Over the years, Godal had developed good links with Brian Greenwood, and while their personal research interests had taken them to different sides of the African continent, this was at a time when the global health community was numerically small and interconnected on a personal level. Brian Greenwood became the custodian of the award and remembers that its acquisition caused some tribulations;

> the first TDR grant was very large, about \$1 million and I got into trouble with MRC Head Office for getting this money, which in those days was a large grant, as the directors of MRC units were not meant to solicit external funds, very different from now.[22]

The Study, Results and Impact

The large trial was run and overseen from Farafenni, which at the time was a relatively isolated town over 100 km from the capital Banjul; the study was well planned and implemented but was beset with unforeseen problems in the days leading up to its launch on 1 July 1989. First, a truly bizarre incident involved the cash payroll that was dispatched once a month from the MRC's base in Fajara to its staff in Farafenni. Following an overnight robbery, the payroll was stolen and in the confusion that followed, the local police in addition to rounding up the usual suspects also arrested the MRC's lab technicians and put them all in jail! Luckily, they were released before their absence jeopardised the trial's launch. Misfortune then supplanted mistaken identity when the hard drive broke on the computer that was going to be used to record the details of the thousands of people taking part in the survey – fortunately a substitute was dispatched by the MRC; and finally, the researchers couldn't find the store of insecticide that was going to be used to treat the nets, and they only got the *permethrin* to the last village at midnight on 30 June.

The Effect of Insecticide-Treated Bed Nets on Mortality of Gambian Children

The cluster randomised trial was large, involving 73 villages on the south bank of the Gambia River with a combined population of 21,157. The demographic surveillance started on 1 July 1988, and deaths in the study villages were recorded and the parents or guardians of the dead children were visited by a field worker who sought their assistance in completing a questionnaire on the causes of the child's death. The 'verbal' or 'oral autopsy' questionnaires were then independently analysed by three doctors and a probable cause of death accepted if agreed by at least two doctors.

A distinctive feature of the trial[23] in The Gambia was its simplicity, and Alonso immersed himself in the study, eagerly awaiting the appearance of the first useful evidence from the experiment.

> After the first year, towards the end of the rainy season, I looked at mortality of the ITN bed nets versus the controls [normal bed nets] and I had to call my friend and colleague Steve Lindsay, the entomologist on the project. I told him, 'Steve, I promise, that I haven't drunk anything strange today, but the results look amazing'. That was the evidence that we published in the *Lancet* paper in 1991. That, I think, it is fair to say, was the turning point for insecticide-treated bed nets![24]

The results of the trial were indeed astonishing, showing a 63% reduction in all-cause mortality among children who slept under treated nets. A common aphorism among medical statisticians is that, 'if a result is too good to be true then it probably *is* too good to be true'. Indeed, the leading tropical epidemiologist, Peter Smith wrote of the results published by Alonso *et al.* in *The Lancet*: 'This remarkable finding was treated with some scepticism as this seemed substantially more deaths than could be attributed to malaria'.[25] What could explain this anomaly? In trying to make sense of a really clear result from a single clinical trial, there is a danger that extrapolation too far may lead to mistaken decisions, but so too may failure to extrapolate far enough. Steve Lindsay understood the magnitude of the trial's findings as a public health measure and offers this explanation of how the 63% reduction in mortality was configured.

> Before, when we interviewed the parents of a dead child to record the symptoms of the fatal illness for the post mortem questionnaires, doctors estimated that 25% of mortality was due to malaria, so then we come along with a 63% reduction – what can explain the difference? The difference is because it is not only malaria that the children are dying of, it was a combination of malaria, diarrhoeal disease and pneumonia, also the children were often malnourished. But if you take one of the big killers away – they survive. The trial was hugely

instructive – the insecticide bed nets that we used were crude but extraordinarily effective.[26]

This evidence was sufficiently persuasive for the Gambian government to initiate a National Insecticide Bednet Programme (NIPB) in 1992 with the objective of introducing this form of malaria control into all large villages in The Gambia.

Unfortunately, the trial was not properly randomised[27] because the intervention and the control groups were not strictly comparable. Although the likelihood of a serious bias as a result of these methodological limitations was small, the researchers themselves advised caution 'before extrapolating our findings to other areas'.[28] Some studies offer the possibility of expanding our understanding of a disease, and others can indicate if one treatment is more efficacious than another, while the most valuable offer insights into how best to prevent a disease. The 1991 experiment seemed to show that a comparatively simple intervention could reduce childhood mortality by two-thirds and constitutes an extraordinary episode in the history of global public health.

When Tore Godal read the findings of the observational study in *The Lancet* in June 1991, he saw the potential significance of insecticide-treated bed nets as a sustainable method of reducing childhood mortality. Nevertheless, when he discussed the trial with his colleague Jacqueline Cattani, director of malaria field research at TDR, he discovered that she was circumspect about the study because of the use of verbal autopsies which she did not think was a precise measure of deaths due to malaria. 'I told Tore', Jackie Cattani recalled from her home in Florida, 'that while there was a role for verbal autopsies we didn't want any ambiguity, and that I did not think the trial produced enough scientific evidence to base a strategy upon'.[29] Cattani was not the only influential person in the WHO malaria community that had misgivings about the study. Jose Najera, Director of the Malaria Action Programme, was, according to Godal, 'wishy-washy and non-committal about bed nets'.[30] This indifference only served to galvanise Godal's efforts to support further phase III trials across Africa where bed net use was uncommon, and transmission rates were high, to see if the reduction in childhood mortality achieved in The Gambia was real and reproducible. Godal was adamant: 'We have to know!'[31] As a scientist, Godal had the ability to question, to innovate and to push projects forward. According to the Swiss epidemiologist Christian Lengeler, there was another important feature to Godal's involvement in the insecticide bed net story:

the Rockefeller Foundation was not really interested in malaria control, and the MRC and Wellcome Trust were involved, but it was TDR who were in that space, and of course Tore was really the one person at the time who had the means to do something about it.[32]

Godal then used all of his considerable diplomatic skill to persuade his TDR colleagues to discontinue other areas of field research and put all available resources into the ITNs, which made an extra US$5 million available. This unprecedented action, according to Cattani, 'took an enormous amount of courage. I was worried about the outcome, and I wasn't sure that insecticide-treated nets would have an impact, but pushing forward with these huge trials in four countries took great vision and bravery'.[33] Godal argued convincingly that a specific intervention, a unique investment, could make a lasting improvement to human health.

The introduction of randomised controlled trials (RCTs) by the UK Medical Research Council in the 1940s constitutes one of the most important experimental advances in modern medicine.[34] If conducted well, the randomised clinical trial is the most powerful and unbiased method of providing accurate and critical evaluations of the efficacy of interventions. Furthermore, accurate data on efficacy allow the calculation of the number of clinical cases or deaths averted by an intervention in a given population. This can be combined with the cost of implementation to obtain cost-effectiveness estimates.[35] Convinced by the dramatic results of the first mortality trial, Godal established a TDR bed net Task Force under Jackie Catanni's direction, to collaborate with other agencies to fund and plan the phase III trials.[36] This consensual attitude aligned with Godal's management style, which rejected sectionalism in favour of consensus; the large randomised controlled trials therefore were not going to be the sole preserve of TDR; instead, they would be co-directed with 20 academic institutions from across the world with proven expertise in tropical disease epidemiology. This collectivist approach was deliberately sought as it had the added benefit of freeing the studies from accusations of predetermination, misconception or bias. Within three months, 10 proposals had been selected by the Task Force, and a workshop was then held in Geneva where the studies were co-developed to allow comparability in analysis. It was crucially important to Godal that investigators on the ground participated in the design of the studies. That then gave them full ownership of the programme, which in turn, Godal believed the studies would be carried out in a better way, rather than if the study design had been developed by one group, far removed from the implementers on the ground. Eventually, four large-scale trials in insecticide-impregnated nets were approved at a cost of US$12 million, in The Gambia, Ghana, Kenya and Burkina Faso,[37] with all-cause child mortality as the principal endpoint, covering a population of nearly 400,000 people. In each of the large trials, there was a significant impact on mortality (ranging from 15% Burkina Faso, 17% Ghana, 25% The Gambia and 33% Kenya) and, although not as great as in the original 1991 study, was nonetheless of profound importance.[38] In 1996, following the completion of the studies, The Malaria Program at WHO immediately announced insecticide-treated bed nets to be a key element in the control of malaria. Yet, even after demonstrating the efficacy, safety and cost-effectiveness of insecticide-impregnated bed nets, to Godal's dismay, it would take almost a decade before the large-scale implementation of this life-saving protection was rolled out across Africa, the world's most malarious continent.

The Forces of Resistance

One of the reasons why insecticide-treated bed nets were not taken up as quickly as they should have been was due, in no small part, to an hypothesis put forward by two leading malaria researchers, Kevin Marsh and Bob Snow.[39] In essence, their theoretical paper postulated: *okay, so you could protect children for a period, but the use of bed nets will only delay their inevitable deaths, because all the intervention is doing is preventing the children from developing immunity. As a consequence, the children just get severe disease at a later stage when they don't use bed nets or drugs or vaccines. There would be a rebound effect.* According to Peter Smith, their paper, 'caused a large debate in the malaria community, because Bob and Kevin were highly respected and I think it made people cautious about the concept of using bed nets'.[40] Kevin Marsh and Bob Snow had worked at the MRC's Laboratories in The Gambia with Brian Greenwood in the 1980s, and even though he recognised that their hypothesis about the impairment of naturally acquired immunity was valid their hypothesis was proved to be wrong.

> Some evidence that rebound malaria has been found with chemoprevention, and perhaps vaccines, but not with ITNs, possibly because the transition from non-protection to protection is more gradual than that seen by drug administration. In the few examples in which 'rebound malaria' has been studied the overall benefits far outreach the subsequent harm.[41]

To Steve Lindsay's mind, the Snow and Marsh paper was 'destructive' and constituted a great deal more than a bit of negative publicity, and it was symptomatic of the wry distain with which the research into the safety and effectiveness of insecticide-impregnated bed nets was viewed within the broader health community. 'People have preconceived ideas and there was a slowness to take up any new intervention', is how Lindsay describes the incompetent scientific doubt about ITNs, 'the old guard entomologists at WHO said "why are we messing around with bed nets? We can do it with indoor residual spraying, we know that works; send the teams in, get the thing done, and then leave"'.[42]

In the wider context of the world of malaria control, there was a metaphysical element at play that clouded judgement and paralysed thinking. The success of Fred L. Soper and the Rockefeller Foundation in eradicating the Anopheles gambiae mosquito from northern Brazil before World War II inspired the ethos of disease eradication into the founding ideals of the newly constituted WHO in April 1948. Seven years later, the first Global Malaria Eradication Programme (GMEP) was launched as the frontline project for the WHO, driven intellectually by a cadre of powerful eradicationalists, who deployed what was believed at the time to be the all-conquering chemical compound DDT and the antimalarial drug chloroquine. It is worth recalling that the first GMEP excluded Africa entirely,

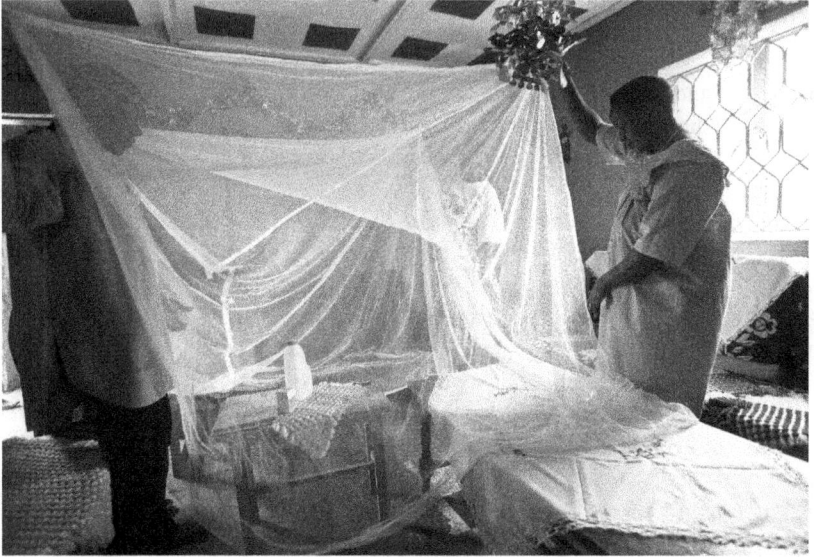

Figure 3.2 Community-Directed Distributors in Uganda, 2007, deliver long-lasting insecticide-treated bed nets (LLITNs). The team is inside a villager's house explaining to the householder (on the right,) how to best hang and use a bed net (which can be used indoors or outdoors).

Source: Courtesy of Andy Crump.

because, in the countries of Sahel and sub-Sahel, transmission levels of the disease were so high it was thought that eradication was impossible until 'conditions were more favourable'. However, increased resistance to DDT led to a resurgence of malaria in many countries and the eradication attempts launched in the 1950s and 1960s ended in failure. Over the following 20 years, the status of malaria research underwent a metamorphosis; from being a pre-eminent WHO frontline priority, to becoming relegated to the status of a *Great Neglected Disease* in 1978 by the Rockefeller Foundation.[43] As a consequence, by the 1980s the malaria control people had more or less given up; the dystopian reality was famously described by Ian McGregor, a former director of the MRC's Gambian field station at Fajara: 'The malaria campaign of the WHO clearly failed to eradicate malaria and merely succeeded in eradicating malariologists and research'.[44] The paradox of the failure of WHO malaria eradication campaign was that it stifled innovation. This contradiction itself formed a decisive moment and was the motivating factor behind Godal's investigations across the entire spectra of public health including drug development and field interventions to find a new strategy for malaria control. As the Director of TDR, Godal saw at first hand the cognitive dissonance that permeated the WHO thinking as a direct result of not learning lessons from the failure of eradication.

> The paradox was that they had their fingers burned, but still the whole strategy of eradication continued running like a machine. . . . It was known that there was parasite resistance to chloroquine but they were afraid to change anything that would increase costs, so they just stayed with it.[45]

In the same way that parasites became resistant to DDT, the WHO had become resistant to change. One of the biggest challenges any institution can face is to change its mental framework. Tragically, the spirit of innovation had been extinguished in the WHO malaria world and replaced by a debilitating reluctance to change behaviour out of fear of repeating another damaging failure. The bureaucratic 'machine' continued to propel a failed strategy into a seemingly endless holding pattern circling high above an Edenic delusion. This atrophying of innovation delayed the adoption of insecticide-treated bed nets that had been shown to reduce all-cause mortality in African children by nearly 20% even in areas of hyperendemic malaria transmission.[46]

Beyond the monolithic obstacle of WHO dogma, the early trials sponsored by TDR were the main impetus for the distribution of insecticide-treated nets in Africa. The advent of the new approach prompted a long-running and damaging debate: should treated nets be distributed free of charge or should recipients make a contribution? Some, like the medical entomologist and long-term advocate of ITNs, Chris Curtis, feared that attempts to sell them might limit their use and so jeopardise the community as against the individual value of the scheme. This was a febrile dispute, occasionally conducted in the corridors of Curtis's home institution, the London School of Hygiene and Tropical Medicine.[47] Curtis had been involved in ITNs technology at every stage, from the basic entomological work, through village-scale trials, to strategies for large-scale implementation.[48] One of Curtis's theories was that if most people in a village used ITNs a 'mass effect' would reduce the entire mosquito population and thereby protect even those without nets. A committed Socialist, Curtis developed this concept into a political argument in favour of 'free nets' – the principle that donor funds should be used to provide treated nets to everyone in areas of high transmission. In the years leading up to the new millennium, the damaging battle continued about how to get the insecticide bed nets to the people that needed them most. Steve Lindsay viewed it as an argument, 'that went on and on forever. It was sapping'.

Putting Economics at the Heart of Global Health

Many factors shape the health of individuals and the great variability of health within and across nations. Indisputably economic status strongly affects human life expectancy, and in the final quarter of the twentieth century moral and numerical arguments increasingly gained traction that emphasised the importance of investments in health as essential components of the economic growth policies that seek to improve the conditions of the poor in low- and middle-income countries. Progressively, the enumeration of mortality, which had happened in a few of the developed countries over the previous century, was expanded to give a more accurate picture of who was dying of what diseases in different populations. This approach marked a turning point: every year, some eight million children in low- and middle-income countries died from just five conditions: pneumonia, diarrhoeal disease, malaria, measles and malnutrition. Almost half of these preventable diseases could be inexpensively prevented or cured; as a consequence, what was called for by some global health researchers was a cost-effective[49] and selective primary health care programme of medical intervention to address this unmet need.[50] The goal was to help the greatest number of people in the most cost-effective manner possible.

The principle of measuring the global burden of disease and the drive to address health inequalities and inefficiencies in global health led to the landmark World Bank's *World Development Report (WDR) 1993: investing in health*.[51] The WDR 1993 was led by the health economist, Dean Jamison, and contained a team including, among others, Christopher Murray and Richard Feachem; this study represented an experimental advance in efforts to systematise the establishment of priorities for the control of the major disease in the developing world. The report used the 'disability-adjusted life year' (DALY) to measure the burden of disease; this enabled the authors to give a cost–benefit analysis without putting a dehumanising value on a human life. As the report stated on its opening page,

> In addition to premature mortality, a substantial portion of the burden of disease consists of disability ranging from polio-related paralysis to blindness to suffering brought about by severe psychosis. To measure the burden of disease, this Report uses the disability-adjusted life year mortality with those lost as a result of disability.[52]

WDR 1993, which Jamison today evaluates as a 'centre left report from a centre right institution'[53] is rightly celebrated as a major contribution to finding the most cost-effective form of medical intervention to help reduce the sequence of exposure, disability and death in the developing world. Because good health increases the economic productivity of individuals and the economic growth rate of countries, the report showed that investing in health is one means of accelerating development. By quantifying the global burden of disease, for the first time it became obvious what the big killers were across humanity; with regard to infectious diseases, malaria was recognised as a huge problem and the most deadly of all the parasitic diseases. The Report, because of its statistical clarity and conceptual originality, did a great deal to catalyse fresh thinking in the global health world. One of the major ideas advocated by Dean Jamison and his colleagues – and for which they received vitriolic criticism[54] – was identifying a role for the private sector in helping to deliver health care programmes. After the report had been written, Jamison was invited to meet with his new boss at the World Bank, Michael Bruno. At the meeting, Bruno said to his colleague, 'You went into this report pretty well knowing what your conclusions were going to be, I bet. I don't want to know what those conclusions were. I want to know what conclusion you came to that wasn't on that list'. Jamison's answer was immediate: 'Scientific advance rather than economic advance, and that the huge changes to human health over the century were a product of technological change'.[55] The recognition that the most important element driving improvements in health was scientific knowledge and its application both in creating powerful interventions and in guiding behaviour was a vindication of Godal's vision for global health. WDR 1993 was a memorable and persuasive study; it produced convincing evidence of the benefits of investing in health, showed that 'the language of economics was important', and crucially, identified policies for improving health in developing countries. For these policies to be implemented, the WHO would need a strategically adept and committed leadership that had the political experience to get things done.

A Call for Change at the World Health Organization

In 1998, the curtain finally came down on Hiroshi Nakajima's tenure as Director-General of the World Health Organization (WHO). Nakajima's decade long custodianship of the WHO had been inauspicious, marred by accusations of vacillation (he shunned the WDP 93 report, even though the WHO was partly responsible for its commissioning), mismanagement and lack of a clear sense of programme direction.[56] Under Nakajima, the WHO had become increasingly emasculated and steadily moved aside not only on the international development scene but also ominously within the health field. Nakajima's successor, Gro Harlem Brundtland, was everything he was not: they were as different as night and day; matter and antimatter. Gro Harlem Brundtland was a widely respected, scientifically literate physician, who had been elected Prime Minister of Norway in 1981 – the youngest person and first woman ever to hold that office. Brundtland was born in Oslo in 1939, and served three terms as Prime Minister of Norway between 1981 and 1996; under her leadership, Norwegian society became internationally identified with social democracy, in its efforts to bring about peace, reconciliation, public health aid and development around the world. In addition, she founded and led the influential UN Commission on the Environment and Development, which was widely referred to as the Brundtland Commission.[57] In April 1987, when the Commission published its report *Our Common Future*, it helped establish the concept of 'sustainable development' which laid the philosophical foundations for the 1992 Earth Summit in Rio de Janeiro.

The combination of being a physician and an internationally respected politician should have led almost inevitably to Brundtland putting herself forward for the election to be the Director-General of the World Health Organization. But as Brundtland revealed in her autobiography, in a passage subtitled *The Persuasive Power of Four Blue Eyes*, she admitted to have more or less been pushed into entering the global electoral race.

> In March [1997] two enthusiastic men had visited my office in the Norwegian Parliament. Both were my colleagues in the medical profession. One of them, Dr Sverre Lie, came from my own class at the Medical Faculty of the University of Oslo. He had specialised in paediatrics and had worked for the WHO on projects in the Middle East. An idealist. A humanist. The other, Dr. Tore Godal, was a specialist in tropical medicine, also from the University of Oslo, who had long worked for the WHO in Ethiopia and as a director in Geneva. They brought one message only: 'Gro, you are the natural next Director General of the World Health Organisation. We really need you. Only you can make a difference. Norway has never had a better candidate for a U.N. position. You can surely win. Please do it. Do it in order to put new life into the most important specialised agency of the United Nations, the significance of which is on the rise because of new and re-emerging diseases'.

'Making a Difference' was the slogan of Brundtland's campaign which was expertly led by her Norwegian political adviser, intellectual heavyweight and Labour Party colleague (and now Prime Minister of Norway) Jonas Gahr Støre. A formidable politician in her own right, Brundtland could feel that there was a mandate for change blowing through the corridors of the WHO in Geneva and she was determined to use this favourable climate to bring about fundamental change in health thinking. On the campaign trail, Brundtland held off soliciting declarations of support from other European countries and instead opted to show the global approach she would bring to the WHO by heading for the continent of Africa. One of Brundtland's electoral advantages was that she was from Norway, a country that had never been a colonial power; in fact, it had itself been a colony under Denmark and Sweden. Thus, there was no negative history to muddy the waters of her idealism. Additionally, since the 1970s, with the establishment of the Armauer Hansen Research Institute in Addis Abba, Ethiopia, Norway had engaged with African country partners in building up primary health services, particularly in Botswana where many Norwegian doctors and nurses worked and trained.[58] When Brundtland and Jonas Gahr Støre travelled to African countries in the fall of 1997, visiting patients' wards and talking to health professionals, health ministers and heads of state she always made sure to ask the question: 'What in your view is the biggest disease burden for Africa, malaria or HIV/AIDS?' 'Somewhat surprisingly', Brundtland later wrote, 'everyone gave the same answer: malaria. The spread of the disease was terrifying, the projections of its influence on life expectancy shocking'.[59] Brundtland, like Godal, together with an increasing number of global health thinkers, held the conviction that improved health fosters development and reduces poverty. Throughout the 1990s, as evidence that poverty was the world's biggest killer, accounting for more than 50% of the annual death toll of 12 million children, it became increasingly apparent that spending on health was not an optional extra, but absolutely essential to the development process.[60] The time was now ripe for the WHO to optimise efforts to combat the diseases of poverty, and a constellation of powerful people had now been assembled around Brundtland that believed societies can be changed and that poverty can be fought. Critically, they had a predetermined programme for global health that would reduce the burden of disease on the world's poorest people.

In May 1998, Brundtland was elected Director-General of the WHO and with his insider knowledge of the machinations of WHO politics, Godal was able to help the new administration to create a streamlined leadership structure and develop a vision for the future of world health together with a strategy for implementing it. From the outset, the goal was to lift health to the top of the political agenda – to do that the WHO needed to become more strategic, if it was going to affect change and influence the hearts and minds of key decision-makers worldwide. The new WHO leadership wanted to be standard bearers of knowledge and intervention, to hit the ground running and to accelerate their speed of momentum. Consequently, it was collectively decided to select two priority projects that mirrored the ambition of the new Director-General of the WHO to make a difference to the global burden of disease in the twenty-first century. From the infectious diseases field, malaria was chosen as a 'Cabinet project' directly under Dr Brundtland, and from the non-communicable diseases spectrum, tobacco was targeted because the epidemic of smoking-related deaths had claimed over 100 million lives in the twentieth century.[61] These two big killers were, according to epidemiologist, Richard Peto 'the ideal pair' to concentrate on if the objective was to prevent premature deaths and to reduce poverty.[62] Both were classical and modern challenges. At the World Health Assembly in 1998, Dr Brundtland called upon the audience to confront an emerging global threat by saying: 'Tobacco should not be advertised, subsidized, or glamorized'.[63] The WHO launched the 'Tobacco Free Initiative', and called for a wide range of partners to hold back the relentless increase in tobacco consumption, reverse the epidemic in smoking-related deaths, and to confront powerful vested interests.[64]

Roll Back Malaria

It is worth remembering that at the end of the twentieth century, malaria was primarily restricted to the tropical and sub-tropical areas of the world, but 50 years before, malaria also affected the temperate world including the United States and countries in Europe. During Brundtland's inaugural speech on 13 May 1998, she declared that: 'Malaria is the single largest disease in Africa and a primary cause of poverty. Every day 3,000 children die from malaria. Every year there are 500 million cases among children and adults'.[65] Brundtland echoed a warning that had been made 100 years before, by members of the Italian parliament who lamented the extent to which, 'this disease reduces the welfare, the human resources and the wealth of the land. There is no other health problem so deeply linked to the prosperity of our country'.[66] Brundtland was both a doctor and a politician, and she shared with her team an abiding belief learned in the combative arena of Norwegian politics, that trust was a prerequisite of public health and political action. Trust was the bedrock upon which global health was to be based and, importantly, donors had to be convinced that aid was used efficiently. More than any other WHO Director-General, before or since, Brundtland was overwhelmingly a political leader; of course, she valued health as a human right, and crucially she had the political expertise that enabled her policies to advance and gain adherents and powerful allies in the global health community. Above all, there needed to be a harmony between words and actions and Brundtland, Godal and Gahr Støre formed the nucleus of a campaign within WHO to resurrect malaria into the global health arena. All three were visionaries, propelled by values of equity and fairness – equally, they were also unwavering rationalists, 'determined to bring others along with them, to persevere and not give up'.[67] They believed that by working together it was possible to achieve impressive results that societies can be changed, and that poverty can be fought.

There was an excitement and energy surrounding Brundtland and her transition team, and she was a vital figure in the malaria story because she had the leadership skills to navigate the politics of a changing and increasingly globalised world.[68] This was a period that witnessed the burgeoning of new public–private partnerships which brought together governments, the private-sector, non-governmental organisations (NGOs) and ultimately the planet's economic behemoths The Group of Eight Industrialised Nations (G8). Godal, being a 'natural born strategist'[69] saw the opportunity to use the WHO as the hub of the wheel, from which other partners radiated out, to form an alliance focused on poverty eradication while at the same time attracting more development money into WHO. By the early summer of 1998, Godal had designed a new science-based approach to malaria control that advocated the use of long-lasting insecticide bed nets. When the 'Roll Back Malaria'[70] (RBM) campaign was announced to the world in 1998, it was supported by the Organisation for African Unity.[71] Importantly, RBM was not a renewed attempt to eradicate the disease – the goal was to reduce malaria deaths by half by 2010.[72]

Roll Back Malaria could not have been launched at a more apposite time. It was able to bring the world together and create a new dynamic for malaria control. This force was so palpable that according to the tropical disease epidemiologist, Christian Lengeler, 'you felt there was a new age breaking, bringing new hope to the world'.[73] In the era of antimalarial drug resistance, people had been losing hope on the continent of Africa, and the future had looked gloomy, but the randomised controlled trials of insecticide bed nets offered a realistic prospect for prevention that was feasible. Out of the dystopia came the realisation that there was something very effective against the disease that could generate money, political interest and change the sociological mind-set, because there was a generation of malariologists who still lived in the shadow of the failure to eliminate malaria in the 1960s. This manifested itself in a reluctance within the malaria community to set ambitious programmes. The RBM campaign helped to dissolve this fear and psychologically shift how people thought about malaria control in the era of insecticide-treated bed nets. For those working in global health today, much can be learnt from seeing how Godal turned ideas into actions that were positive. Godal's methods could be viewed as unconventional, in that he was not the loud interventionist type; he preferred anonymity to fame and often said that 'if you want to achieve anything of importance in global health it is better to keep a low profile'.[74] Nor did he deliver grandiloquent lectures, or write long esoteric books; instead, he was renowned for concise, lapidary statements and perceptive insights that provided solutions to complex global health problems that were scientifically eloquent, understandable and persuasive. Concrete outcomes that are easy to communicate were always his objective. Roll Back Malaria was a break with the past; it was a public–private partnership and with Tore Godal as its first Chief Executive, it relaunched and re-energised malaria research and brought the world together following two decades of stagnation.

Global Health and the New Millennium

The forces of change that had been nascent within global health at the end of the twentieth century experienced a great acceleration of unprecedented magnitude in the opening decades of the new millennium. In a way that would have been unthinkable to Halfdan Mahler or even the most optimistic tropical disease researchers in the 1980s, global health became the most innovative forum of international cooperation, overshadowing both the campaign for universal nuclear disarmament and the climate emergency. The era of rapid progress and inventiveness was marked by a concurrence of some key framework conditions that lead to two decades where health outperformed other sectors in terms of inventiveness and demonstrable results. The forces that shaped these changes were in part material, technological and political; some emerged over time, some represented aberrant breakthroughs in thinking and alliances, while others, as in the story of malaria control, illustrate the fascinating nature of having the right constellation of people working together.

The modern history of malaria control is a story of synchronicity, of meaningful coincidences that pulsed forward in time with dramatic effect. The new century witnessed a transformation in global health thinking with the publication of the United Nations Eight Millennium Development Goals (MDGs); this manifesto for change was to be achieved by 2015 and was supported by all of the 191 UN member states. One of the eight goals focused on a pledge 'to combat HIV/AID, malaria, and other diseases', while another underscored a commitment 'to eradicate extreme poverty and hunger'. Collectively, the eight MDGs reflected a growing acknowledgment that the most economically effective way to combat poverty was through better health-led development.[75]

With the announcement of the MDGs, the wider malaria community seized the moment and organised The African Summit on Roll Back Malaria in Abuja, Nigeria on 25 April 2000 – this became an important date in the history of global health: 25 April became World Malaria Day. At the meeting, a new pledge was made to halve malaria deaths by 2010 by implementing the strategies of the RBM programme: ensuring that people had access to insecticide-treated bed nets and chemoprevention (for the prevention of malaria in pregnancy). The Abuja meeting proved a watershed moment in the history of malaria; it no longer occupied the status of a neglected tropical disease, and the presence of more than 30 heads of state was testament to the growing acceptance by the rich countries of the world that their focus should be more clearly on global health and development issues. Brundtland, and her team, who had been in the vanguard of the movement to raise awareness of the catastrophic effects of the disease, attended the Abuja summit and lobbied the political delegations to have malaria, and the wider subject of global health, put on the agenda of the G8 summit due to take place in July, in Okinawa, Japan. But before Brundtland left Abuja, she attended a lecture given by the US economist, Jeffrey Sachs, one of the world's leading experts on sustainable development and poverty. Nina Munk, in her well-conceived and nuanced book *The Idealist: Jeffrey Sachs and the Quest to End Poverty*, describes how Sachs likes to say that malaria represents the great divide between rich and poor.

> Illustrating the point to his students, he superimposes two colour-coded maps: a map of the world's poorest countries, and a map of countries with the highest burden of malaria. With few exceptions, the coloured zones on both maps are nearly identical. The poorer the country, the more likely it is that its people will suffer from malaria.[76]

Sachs was something of a rarity in the field of macroeconomics; he was evangelical about ending global poverty and advocated the free distribution of insecticide-treated bed nets to prevent the spread of malaria. Brundtland was deeply affected by Jeffrey Sachs's lecture and was

> struck by the enormous damage caused by this ancient disease. . . . Short-term economic benefits from malaria control can be up to $12 billion each year. These are staggering numbers and there is no doubt that malaria is taking a big bite out of Africa's economic growth.[77]

A short time later, and acting on the advice of her 'chef du cabinet' Jonas Gahr Støre, Brundtland appointed Sachs to chair the WHO 'Commission on Macroeconomics and Health: investing in health for economic development'. This was a bold appointment and when the Commission's report was published in December 2001, its findings boosted the financial underpinnings of malaria control and contributed to positioning health at the apex of the politics of development.[78]

Meanwhile, the Ghanaian diplomat, Kofi Annan, who had been elected Secretary-General of the United Nations in 1997, was campaigning for a Global Fund to be established, undergirded by a financial 'war chest' to respond to the HIV/AIDS crisis and other infectious diseases that were a disproportionate burden on the world's poor. Originally, discussions had been centred on establishing a Global Fund only for HIV/AIDS, but steadily a consensus began to cohere within a powerful group of global health actors that the parameters of the Global Fund should be widened to encompass TB and malaria. There was a growing momentum around the idea that investing in health was an economically sound way of reducing poverty. The changing alchemical nature of the politics of health reached another high watermark in the summer of 2000 when the G8 summit was held in Okinawa, Japan. For the first time, global health was put on the agenda for discussion. If Godal was a champion of malaria control, then the Japanese public health doctor, Arata Kochi, was the belligerent figure determined to establish tuberculosis as a 'global emergency'. Kochi, in his leadership of the WHO's tuberculosis programme not only made headlines but also concentrated minds by depicting the devastating impact of the disease and promoting the memorably named DOTS (Directly observed treatment, short course) strategy as the most cost-effective way of stopping the disease. In parallel to the growing acceptance of the macroeconomic logic of investing in health to reduce levels of poverty, the influence of a WHO group led by Jonas Gahr Støre began to crystallise around the idea of a massive effort against the three infectious diseases: HIV/AIDS, malaria and tuberculosis.[79] This idea proved attractive to the Japanese hosts of the G8 meeting in Okinawa as the country had a proud history of eliminating malaria and tuberculosis.[80] Consequently, a Global Fund for HIV/AIDS, malaria and TB was adopted in 2000 and formally launched early in 2002. Its first Executive Director was Richard Feachem, and it rapidly became the world's largest health financial institution for developing countries with assets, over three years of US$11 billion. One of the Global Fund's cornerstone programmes was the procurement and distribution of insecticide-treated bed nets. As a result, mortality from malaria dropped steadily in the following years and by 2015 it had more than halved with about 70% of that reduction due to the use of bed nets.

Looking back, it becomes clear that if Roll Back Malaria had not been in existence, the disease would not have been part of the Global Fund, and of crucial importance too was Gro Harlem Brundtland's role in getting Jeffrey Sachs to lead the WHO 'Commission on Macroeconomics and Health'. 'People argue about this, what was the real trigger for the Global Fund, and I don't know if it will ever be settled', believes Richard Horton,

> but it was a truly decisive moment. Jeff will say it was his commission. The Japanese will say it was something they did, and I don't know what the right answer is, but there is no question that Jeff's commission gave the macroeconomic case for why the Global Fund was the right thing to do. The fact that Gro Brundtland got a star economist to lead the commission, that was what made the difference. If it had been a World Health report it wouldn't have had the same credibility, so having an economist was absolutely decisive.[81]

The Global Fund announced a new era in medicine; there was no doubt that medical research had become global, transcending national and geographical boundaries.

Thirty years ago, Steven Lindsay was the entomologist on the original path-breaking study of the efficacy of insecticide-treated bed nets in The Gambia which is now seen as the catalyst for a scientific and political chain reaction

PROTECTIVE EFFECT OF BEDNETS AGAINST EPISODES OF MALARIA IN GAMBIAN CHILDREN

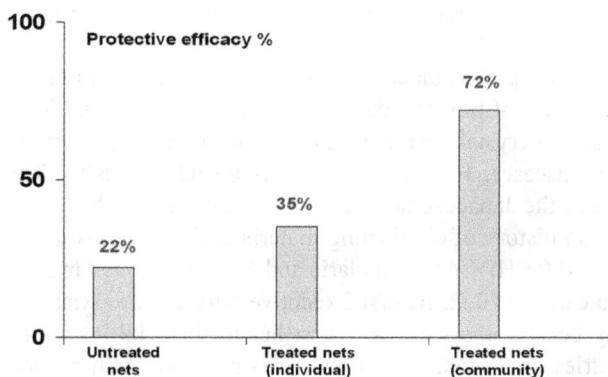

(Snow et al.,1987. TRSTMH; 81:563
Snow et al., 1988. TRSTMH. 82:212 & 838)

Figure 3.3 This graph shows persuasive evidence that insecticide-treated bed nets offered protection to Gambian children from being bitten by a malaria-infected female anopheline mosquito. As most mosquitoes feed at night, sleeping under insecticide-treated bed nets reduces both morbidity and mortality.

Source: Courtesy of Brian Greenwood.

that during the 15-year span of the MDGs led to a remarkable and widespread reduction in the mortality and morbidity caused by malaria in Africa. Lindsay feels that the transformation has been nothing short of 'extraordinary' during his lifetime.

> Because when I was working in the Gambia in the early days, you were used to every child having malaria during the rainy season, there was this appalling mortality rate that you expected to be the same in perpetuity. And to think that when we were there in the late 1980s, 80% of the children had malaria and now probably it is 1% in the general population – that is just extraordinary.[82]

A recent study estimated that *Plasmodium falciparum* infection prevalence in Africa halved and the incidence of clinical disease fell by 40% between 2000 and 2015. The researchers estimated that interventions had averted 663 million clinical cases since 2000, with 'insecticide-treated nets, the most widespread intervention the largest contributor (68% of cases averted)'.[83] When measured by such compelling public health metrics, it is easy to understand why the group of 12 researchers that carried out the original 1991 trial might view the study as a decisive moment in malaria control. Indeed as Lindsay remembers: 'Pedro once said to me, "we will never do anything as good again – and he was right"'.[84]

It had been a long time coming, but Godal had never doubted the science that underpinned the initial cluster randomised controlled trial that he had funded in The Gambia in 1991, and the four subsequent very large RCTs across Africa. These studies helped to change the mind-set of malariologists and activists in the field who were looking for a sustainable way of refocusing the world's attention on preventing the transmission of malaria, which for millennia had been a scourge on the health and economic well-being of millions of the world's poorest people. He was also clear in his own mind why it had taken so long between the trials showing the efficacy and cost-effectiveness of insecticide-treated bed nets and their use by affected communities.

> To me it was simple. The main factor was that financing to distribute nets free of charge only became available with the establishment of the Global Fund. In addition, the availability of long-lasting nets, which do not require re-impregnation made them simpler to apply from an operational point of view.[85]

History has shown that Godal and Jeff Sachs were correct, and we've seen that the free model has allowed for much broader distribution of bed nets – and much greater reductions in malaria – than market models.

Tore Godal successfully guided the Roll Back Malaria programme through the difficult early stages of its inception before handing the organisation to its first executive director, David Nabarro in 1999. Nabarro, who later succeeded Jonas Gahr Støre as Gro Brundtland's 'chef du cabinet', admired Godal's ability to conceive an idea, see it implemented and then deliberately evanesce. 'That' according to Nabarro

> is the whole secret of Tore Godal. He can excite a lot of people about an idea, sketch it out in enough detail so that you can visualise it, and then in an incredibly light touch way, make it easy for it to happen. That is what he did in so many areas of global health. He has worked out in life that if you want something to happen, you crate platforms on which others can take credit, and you don't demand any credit for it yourself. His whole personality is based on not needing accolades. He has been able to transform so many areas by this capacity to let others get on with things – and then he just walks away.[86]

In 1999, Godal's long career within the highest echelons of world health appeared to be coming to an end as his 60th birthday – the mandatory retirement for all WHO personnel – rapidly approached. Retirement at 60 had been an inviolable policy change brought in by Brundtland's administration, but surely, for Godal an exception would be made . . . No dispensation was sought and nor was it offered. Later that year, Godal found himself under the shadow of a low-level depression in an IKEA showroom, selecting the office furniture for his reincarnation as 'global health consultant'. As he contemplated the merits of an equipoise reading lamp, his phone rang. It was Tim Evans, Director of the Rockefeller Foundation in New York. He said that there was a new US philanthropist on the block named Bill Gates, in the tradition of John D. Rockefeller, and would Tore be willing to engage in a new vaccine initiative? After the call, Godal turned on his heels and left the showroom.

Notes

1. G. Brundtland, *Madam Prime Minister: A Life in Power and Politics* (New York: Farrar, Straus and Giroux, 2002), p. 462.
2. M. Gillies, *Mayfly on the Stream of Time* (London: Message Books, 2000).
3. K. Marsh, "Malaria disaster in Africa", *Lancet*, 1998, 352, pp. 924–925.
4. S. W. Lindsay, M. E. Gibson, "Bed nets revisited: Old idea, new angle", *Parasitology Today*, 1988, 4, pp. 270–272.
5. C. Lengeler, R. W. Snow, "From efficacy to effectiveness: Insecticide treated bed nets in Africa", *Bulletin of the World Health Organisation*, 1996, 74 (3), pp. 325–332.
6. W. R. Ballou et al., "Safety and efficacy of a recombinant DNA *Plasmodium falciparum* sporozoite vaccine", *Lancet*, 6 June 1987, 1 (8545), pp. 1277–1281.
7. Interview with Brian Greenwood, May 2016.
8. Brian Greenwood, personal email communication, April 2020.
9. R. W. Snow et al., "Permethrin-treated bed nets (mosquito nets) prevent malaria in Gambian children", *Transactions of the Royal Society of Tropical Medicine and Hygiene*, 1988, 82, pp. 838–842.
10. R. W. Snow et al., "Permethrin-treated bed nets (mosquito nets) prevent malaria in Gambian children", *Transactions of the Royal Society of Tropical Medicine and Hygiene*, 1988, 82, pp. 838–842.

11. World Health Organization, *The Use of Impregnated Bed Nets and Other Materials for Vector-Borne Disease Control: A Report of the WHO/VBC Informal Consultation held in Geneva, 14–18 February 1989* (Geneva: World Health Organization, 1989).

12. Interview with Pedro Alonso, November 2019.

13. Interview with Steven Lindsay, June 2020.

14. Interview with Steven Lindsay, June 2020.

15. Interview with Pedro Alonso, November 2019.

16. World Health Organization, *The Use of Impregnated Bed Nets and Other Materials for Vector-Borne Disease Control: A Report of the WHO/VBC Informal Consultation held in Geneva, 14–18 February 1989* (Geneva: World Health Organization, 1989), p. 29.

17. World Health Organization, *The Use of Impregnated Bed Nets and Other Materials for Vector-Borne Disease Control: A Report of the WHO/VBC Informal Consultation held in Geneva, 14–18 February 1989* (Geneva: World Health Organization, 1989), p. 29.

18. The primary health care programme was introduced in 1983 in an attempt to establish low-cost, community-based health programmes in low-income countries. An important part of the programme in the Farafenni area was the identification and training of a Traditional Birth Attendant in each village with a population of 400 or greater. In addition, every five villages shared a paid Community Health Nurse.

19. D. Rowe, "The special programme for research and training in tropical diseases", in R. K. Chandra (ed.), *Critical Reviews in Tropical Medicine*, vol. 2 (Boston: Springer, 1984), pp. 1–38.

20. R. Lane, "Profile: Tore Godal: Quiet colossus of global health", *Lancet*, 2019, 394 (10215), p. 2142.

21. T. Godal, "Fighting the parasites of poverty: Public research, private industry and tropical diseases", *Science*, 24 June 1994, 264 (5167), pp. 1864–1866.

22. Brian Greenwood, personal email communication, June 2020.

23. P. L. Alonso, S. W. Lindsay, J. R. M. Armstrong, A. de Francisco, F. C. Shenton, B. M. Greenwood, M. Conteh, M. K. Cham, A. G. Hill, P. H. David, G. Fegan, A. J. Hall, "The effect of insecticide treated bed nets on mortality of Gambian children", *Lancet*, 1991, 337, pp. 1499–1502.

24. Interview with Pedro Alonso, November 2019.

25. Interview with Peter Smith, December 2019.

26. Interview with Steve Lindsay, May 2020.

27. C. Lengeler, J. Armstrong-Schellenberg, U. D'Alessandro, F. Binka, J. Cattani, "Relative versus absolute risk of dying reduction after using insecticide-treated nets for malaria control in Africa", *Tropical Medical and Environmental Health*, 1998, 3 (4), pp. 286–290.

28. P. L. Alonso, S. W. Lindsay, J. R. M. Armstrong, A. de Francisco, F. C. Shenton, B. M. Greenwood, M. Conteh, M. K. Cham, A. G. Hill, P. H. David, G. Fegan, A. J. Hall, "The effect of insecticide treated bed nets on mortality of Gambian children", *Lancet*, 1991, 337, pp. 1499–1502.

29. Interview with Jacqueline Cattani, June 2020.

30. Interview with Tore Godal, November 2019.

31. Interview with Jacqueline Cattani, June 2020.

32. Interview with Christian Lengeler, July 2020.

33. Interview with Jacqueline Cattani, June 2020.

34. C. Keating, "Introducing a history of key trials in the Lancet", *Lancet*, 2017, 390, p. 2025.

35. C. Lengeler, R. W. Snow, "From efficacy to effectiveness: Insecticide treated bed nets in Africa", *Bulletin of the World Health Organization*, 1996, 74 (3), p. 326.

36. The Canadian International Development Agency (CIDA), the International Development Research Centre (IDRC), the United Nations Children's Fund (UNICEF), the UK Overseas Development Agency (ODA), the Danish International Development Agency (DANIDA), the Wellcome Trust, the UK Medical Research Council (MRC), the African Medical Research Foundation (AMREF), the London School of Hygiene and Tropical Medicine (LSHTM), Action Aid The Gambia (AAG), Save the Children Federation (SCFUSA), the Christian Children's Fund (CCF), the Kenyan Medical Research Institute (KEMRI), as well as various national ministries of health (MOHs).
37. Because of the extreme heat in Burkina Faso, insecticide impregnated mesh 'curtains' were used instead of nets.
38. In Burkina Faso, because of the very hot climate, insecticide-treated 'curtains' were used instead of bed nets, which were positioned in front of doors and windows.
39. R. W. Snow, K. Marsh, "Will reducing P. falciparum transmission alter malaria mortality among African children?", *Parasitology Today*, 1995, 11 (5), pp. 188–190.
40. Interview with Peter Smith, December 2019.
41. Brian Greenwood, personal email communication.
42. Interview with Steven Lindsay, May 2020.
43. C. Keating, *Kenneth Warren and the Great Neglected Diseases of Mankind Programme: The Transformation of Geographical Health in the US and Beyond* (New York: Springer, 2017).
44. Interview with Pedro Alonso, November 2019.
45. Interview with Tore Godal, November 2019.
46. C. Lengeler, "Insecticide-treated bed nets and curtains for preventing malaria", *Cochrane Database Systematic Review*, 2004, (2), p. CD000363.
47. Interview with Brian Greenwood, May 2016.
48. C. F. Curtis et al., "Impregnated bed nets and curtains against malaria mosquitoes", in C. F. Curtis (ed.), *Control of Disease Vectors in the Community* (London: Wolfe, 1991), pp. 5–46.
49. S. B. Halstead, J. A. Walsh, K. S. Warren (eds.), *Good Health Care at Low Cost: Proceedings of a Conference at the Bellagio Conference Centre, Italy. 29 April–3 May* (New York: Rockefeller Foundation, 1985). The publication followed a meeting at Bellagio organised by Kenneth S. Warren to bring together demographers, economists and epidemiologists to examine why it was that some countries provided better health care than others while having similar levels of health expenditure.
50. J. A. Walsh, K. S. Warren, "Selective primary health care: An interim strategy for disease control in developing countries", *New England Journal of Medicine*, 1979, pp. 967–974.
51. *World Development Report 1993: Investing in Health* (New York: OUP, 1993).
52. *World Development Report 1993: Investing in Health* (New York: OUP, 1993), p. 1.
53. Interview with Dean Jamison, February 2020.
54. R. Lane, "Profile of Dean Jamison: Putting economics at the heart of global health", *Lancet*, 2013, 382, p. 1871.
55. Interview with Dean Jamison, February 2020.
56. M. Douglas, "Hiroshi Nakajima, leader of W.H.O., dies at 84", *The New York Times*, 28 January 2013.
57. In the Foreword to the report, published by Oxford University Press, Gro Harlem Brundtland wrote 'the "environment" is where we all live; and "development" is what we do in attempting to improve our lot within that abode. The two are inseparable. Further, development issues must be seen as crucial by the political leaders who feel that their countries have reached a plateau towards which other nations must strive. Many of the development paths of the industrialized nations are clearly

unsustainable. And the development decisions of these countries, because of their great economic and political power, will have a profound effect upon the ability of all people's to sustain human progress for generations to come'.

58. Interview with Jonas Gahr Støre, May 2019.
59. G. Brundtland, *Madam Prime Minister: A Life in Power and Politics* (New York: Farrar, Straus and Giroux, 2002), p. 462.
60. WHO, *World Health Report: Making a Difference* (Geneva: WHO, 1999).
61. R. Peto, "Smoking and death: The past 40 years and the next 40", *British Medical Journal*, 1994, 309, pp. 337–339.
62. Interview with Richard Peto, May 2018.
63. G. Brundtland, *Madam Prime Minister: A Life in Power and Politics* (New York: Farrar, Straus and Giroux, 2002), p. 463.
64. In 1999, global tobacco was made a priority of WHO, and work began on the WHO Framework Convention on Tobacco Control. In August 2022, a Global Burden of Disease study published in The *Lancet* showed that, 'smoking remained the leading risk factor for risk-attributable cancer burden'.
65. G. Brundtland, World Health Organization, Speech to the Fifty-First World Health Assembly. May 13 1998, A51/DIV/6, p. 6.
66. The members of the Italian Parliament Giustino Fortunato and Leopoldo Franchette in their circular letter to sponsor the Societa Italiana per gli Studi della Malaria. July 14 1889.
67. Interview with David Nabarro, August 2020.
68. Interview with Richard Horton, August 2020.
69. Interview with Jonas Gahr Støre, April 2019.
70. The name Roll Back Malaria came from Jonas Gahr Støre's children. Jonas tested various names out with his children over breakfast and Roll Back Malaria became the nomenclature of a WHO lodestar programme.
71. From the mid-1990s, a parallel important movement developed in Africa named Africa Initiative for Malaria (AIM) which coincided with WHO's RBM campaign – AIM's message was 'we need to use existing tools better, and we need a systems approach to delivery'. AIM and RBM showed a united front, and AFRO decided to convert AIM to RBM in the Africa region.
72. D. N. Nabarro, E. M. Taylor, "The roll back malaria campaign", *Science*, 26 June 1998, 280, pp. 2067–2068.
73. Interview with Christian Lengeler, July 2020.
74. Interview with Tore Godal, August 2018.
75. D. E. Bloom, D. Canning, "The health and wealth of nations", *Science*, 18 February 2000, 287 (5456), pp. 1207–1209.
76. N. Munk, *The Idealist: Jeffrey Sachs and the Quest to End Poverty* (New York: Doubleday 2013), p. 93.
77. G. Brundtland, *Madam Prime Minister: A Life in Power and Politics* (New York: Farrar, Straus and Giroux, 2002), p. 462.
78. According to Godal, Jeff Sachs visited WHO in the autumn of 1998 and gave a fantastic seminar on the impact of malaria on economic development. This established the relationship between Gro Brundtland and Jonas Gahr Støre and led to the idea of a Commission on Macroeconomics and Health which crystallised during 1999. Gro Brundtland had the idea of a commission, a first in global health, based on her experience of the Brundtland Commission.
79. Dr Brundtland had been invited to Tokyo in the spring of 2000 as part of the preparations for the G8 Summit. In Tokyo, Dr Brundtland presented arguments for The Fund, focusing on the three diseases, rather than just HIV/AIDS.

80. In March 2014, Russia was suspended indefinitely following the annexation of Crimea, whereupon the political forum reverted to G7.
81. Interview with Richard Horton, August 2020.
82. Interview with Steven Lindsay, June 2020.
83. S. Bhatt, D. J. Weiss, E. Cameron, D. Bisanzio, B. Mappin et al., "The effect of malaria control on plasmodium falciparum in Africa between 2000 and 2015", *Nature*, 2015, 526 (7572), pp. 207–211.
84. Interview with Steven Lindsay, June 2020.
85. Interview with Tore Godal, August 2018.
86. Interview with David Nabarro, August 2020.

4 GAVI

The Vaccine Alliance in the Twenty-First Century

Tore Godal is a big ideas person. What he is very good at is seeing the big picture, and he is made of steel in terms of his grit and determination to get things done.

Richard Horton[1]

On 31 January 2000, the Global Alliance for Vaccines and Immunisation (GAVI) was inaugurated at the World Economic Forum in Davos, Switzerland; the high-profile launch being made possible by a large benefaction from the Bill and Melinda Gates Foundation. GAVI brought together a powerful coalition that included UN agencies, governments, the vaccine industry and civil society that within a generation revolutionized efforts to protect the world's poorest children from some of the most deadly infectious diseases. Therefore, GAVI's achievements form a critical chapter in the long history of the influence of vaccination campaigns on public health that had begun with Edward Jenner's introduction of a smallpox vaccine in 1796. The eradication of smallpox in 1979 constitutes a great human accomplishment because smallpox was a universally feared disease, which killed almost 300 million people in the twentieth century alone.[2] Moreover, eradication came as a direct result of the successful collaboration of politics and biomedical science in the form of an adequately financed and inventively led Smallpox Eradication Programme, directed by the WHO. In little more than a decade, the viral disease that had decimated human populations for over 3,000 years[3] was eradicated in every country of the world. This universality, for the first time, led governments, UN institutions, medical science and philanthropic agencies to think in terms of *global health*. This historic success laid the foundation for subsequent global immunisation campaigns for polio, measles, hepatitis and the use of other combination vaccines against diphtheria, pertussis (whooping cough) and tetanus. By the 1980s, while the overall status of immunisation was on an upward trajectory with the science of vaccinology making key advances, there remained a troubling and long time lag between the introduction of a vaccine in wealthy industrialised countries and its use in poorer countries, where death rates were far greater. Traditionally, there was a 20-year

DOI: 10.4324/9781003363859-5

delay between the development of vaccines for the children of the industrialised countries and their availability at prices low enough that they could be bought for the children of low-income countries.[4] During this long interval, millions of poor children in the Global South died from contracting infectious diseases while the children of the richer countries were immunised. Finding cost-effective ways to increase worldwide access to childhood vaccines, thereby avoiding millions of preventable deaths, has been a major endeavour of the global health community over the past 40 years.

A Clash of Health Philosophies and the Modern History of Immunisation Before GAVI

The ideological differences concerning the most effective ways to treat and prevent the major health problems in low-income countries originate from two highly influential nineteenth-century medical researchers, Sir Patrick Manson and Sir Ronald Ross. The work of Manson and Ross helped to establish 'tropical medicine' as a discipline concerned, in the main, with infectious diseases – later the terms 'international' or 'geographical'[5] medicine gained traction before being superseded by 'global medicine' in the last quarter of the twentieth century. As with other spheres of human endeavour, the ever-changing world of medical science has produced divergent philosophies and opposing schools of thought that have propagated adherents, devotees and dissenters. Some of these theories, in both the tropical medicine and global health era, have occupied semi-divine status, provoked bitter and long-lasting turf wars or caused personal relationships, as between Manson and Ross, to be troubled and at times neuralgic. The accumulated observations made by Manson and Ross while conducting medical research led them to develop contradictory principles about the causes and treatment of disease that later divided into two opposing camps. Patrick Manson, a bank manager's son from Aberdeen, where he studied medicine, discovered the mosquito transmission of filariasis – the cause of elephantiasis – in Amoy, China, in the 1870s. He believed that the attainment of good health for the European colonisers of nations with tropical climates lay in the scientific findings made in the laboratory. In the 1898 preface to his book, *Tropical Diseases: A Manual of the Diseases of Warm Climates*, he described the imperial way forward:

> I now firmly believe in the possibility of tropical colonisation by the white races. Heat and moisture are not in themselves the direct causes of any important tropical disease. The direct causes of 99% of these diseases are germs. To kill them is simply a matter of knowledge.

In contrast, Ross, a Nobel Prize winner for discovering that the mosquito was the vector for malaria, took a more holistic approach to the absence of disease and the ambrosia of wellness, the vital elements of which were 'general living conditions, diet, and sanitation as the main determinants of health'. This marked the beginning of a polarization of approaches to health in the less developed world that still persisted when Tore Godal started his long career in global health. By the early part of the twentieth century, the Manson and Ross methodologies had distilled into the so-called vertical approaches – direct, targeted programmes using specific technologies such as drugs, vaccines and insecticides – and 'horizontal' approaches, which simultaneously used all means – medical, ecological, sociological and political – to improve health. During the formative early decades of the last century, the vertical strategy gained ascendancy.

From the 1950s onwards, the WHO's large-scale vertical eradication programmes were dominated by the campaigns against tuberculosis and yaws (a bacterial disease of the skin and bones) which typified the approach that Patrick Manson had outlined, and some initial success made it an exemplar for a more ambitious undertaking: the eradication of malaria. As we recorded in the previous chapter, that eradication effort, begun in 1955, collapsed in dystopian disarray in the 1970s. The failure to fulfil the promise to eradicate malaria led to a wholesale revolt – not from the poor who were increasingly subject to the ravages of the diseases but from some elements within the scientific community and the WHO in particular against the strategy of disease eradication and the vertical approach in particular. Disenchantment was so great that even the unprecedented success of the Smallpox Eradication Programme had little effect in rehabilitating the centrality of biomedical science to health amelioration.

Unsurprisingly, with so many diseases being manifestations of poverty, horizontal approaches became more prominent as the backlash developed. Battle lines were drawn and intellectual wagons circled. In the period from 1965 to the early 1980s, many within the institutions of world health saw socio-economic development as an answer to the entire developing world's diseases. The change in emphasis corresponded to the reconfiguration of agencies that were the custodians of the world's most vulnerable populations. With some three billion people in those countries suffering from infectious diseases, it was imperative to reduce the sequence of exposure, disability and death. The abandonment of the disease-targeted, vertical approach led to a preoccupation with primary health care, defined 'in its original and narrowest sense (as) frontline or first-contact care, where people meet health workers'.[6]

The doctrine of comprehensive primary health care was nurtured by the charismatic Halfdan T. Mahler, a Danish physician, appointed the Director-General of WHO in May 1973. Under Mahler's leadership, the WHO experienced a metamorphosis, a philosophical redirection away from curative towards preventive care.[7] Viscerally he saw that the most productive way forward was to jettison the white heat of medical technology promoted by some physicians and bureaucrats, and embrace the ideal of primary health workers based on the illustrious barefoot doctors of 1920s China. An opportunity to realise his vision occurred in September 1978, when the International Conference on Primary Health Care was held at Alma-Ata, then the capital of the Soviet Republic of Kazakhstan. The six-day meeting was jointly sponsored by the WHO and UNICEF and was attended by 3,000 delegates from 134 governments across the world. The culmination of the ambitious conference was the production of the Declaration of Alma-Ata, which enshrined health as 'a fundamental human right'. The means of achieving this commendable aim was through comprehensive primary health care, which was defined as being

> the attainment by all peoples of the world by the year 2000 of a level of health that will permit them to lead a socially and economically productive life. From the outset, the declaration of Alma-Ata was seen by some as noble and portentous and by others as utopian and contentious.[8]

However, Mahler was not alone in wanting to redesign the intellectual landscape of global health. In 1980, James 'Jim' Grant became the executive director of the United Nation's International Children's Emergency Fund (UNICEF). Dynamic and charming, Grant had been deeply influenced by the work of his father, John Grant, the medical missionary who had pioneered the training of the barefoot doctors in China that Mahler so admired. In his role at UNICEF, Grant pledged to reduce the suffering and increase the well-being of the world's children, but how was this to be achieved at a time when the developing world was experiencing a major economic recession caused by yet another oil crisis? The answer for Grant lay in prevention along the lines of the low-cost, high-impact vertical targeted interventions that influential Rockefeller Foundation researchers advocated.[9] Under Grant's leadership, UNICEF retreated from a holistic approach to primary health care, and in 1983, he made a decisive move declaring 'A Children's Revolution' focusing solely on universal childhood immunisation. Grant and Mahler – and their respective UN organisations – now held opposing views; they were both idealist, determined to succeed, and set on a collision course.

An internecine turf war that seemed imminent was avoided by the subtle mediation skills of William 'Bill' Foege, one of the highly respected smallpox eradication pioneers. There was much to play for; in the late 1970s, the US through a combination of political commitment, trained staff and well-funded programmes had achieved immunisation rates of over 90% against a variety of preventable childhood diseases. Meanwhile, the WHO's Expanded Programme on Immunisation (EPI) languished, with less than 5% of children in the developing world receiving vaccines; even the traditional vaccines, such as DPT (diphtheria, pertussis, tetanus), were reaching only a small percentage of children.[10] These were the socio-medical forces that brought together powerful individuals and institutions, including Jonas Salk, developer of the world's first polio vaccine, the World Bank and the Rockefeller Foundation to mobilise a new endeavour – universal childhood immunisation by 1990. Many obstacles would need to be overcome if success was to be achieved because the EPI was starved of resources, lacked cohesion, and most debilitating of all was that a spirit of competition rather than cooperation existed between the WHO and UNICEF. In what Bill Foege has described as an act of 'ego suppression', Mahler and Grant visited him in Atlanta for what turned out to be an extraordinary conversation.

> There was just the two of them, and for a while I believed that I was a therapist because they told me that 'we both have such big egos that we sometimes have trouble getting along'. Because it is always hard to get groups to work together who cherish their own turf.[11]

Foege's emollient diplomacy helped to persuade Grant and Mahler to bury their own differences and act with urgency and common purpose to improve the health of the poorest children; this in turn led to a historic meeting at the Rockefeller Foundation's Bellagio conference centre in Italy on 12–16 March 1984. The meeting launched *The Task Force for Child Survival and Development*, and under the direction of Bill Foege the concept of universal childhood immunization was seriously embraced. Over the next six years, immunisation rates increased rapidly from 5% to over 60% in some of the world's lowest income countries – a remarkable achievement.[12]

Despite this astonishing progress, nearly 30 million children in developing countries still did not receive the basic recommended vaccines, leading to more than four million children dying every year from vaccine-preventable diseases. By the end of the 1990s, the Children's Vaccine Initiative, after almost a decade in operation, had failed to build on the achievements of the past: vaccine coverage had stagnated, collaborative programmes with the vaccine industry withered, and most damaging of all, it did not have the trust of the WHO. In March 1998, immunization coverage had slipped to dismal levels in many countries,[13] and this seeming indifference by the wealthy nations to vaccinating the poor[14] led to a high-powered meeting of UN agencies, and the vaccine industry at the World Bank in Washington, DC. Gro Harlem Brundtland attended this meeting, and as the goal of the WHO 'is the vaccination of every child'; she called for the development of new vaccines against HIV/AIDS, malaria and tuberculosis. In their defence, the vaccine-producing companies countered that before the public sector demand new vaccines, they should first systematically roll out the ones that already existed. They had a point. At the time, vaccines were available that were not reaching those people most in need of them. Hepatitis B vaccine was a case in point, killing more than 900,000 people a year, the majority in poor countries. Similarly, Haemophilus influenza type B, or Hib, was one of the biggest vaccine-preventable causes of death in under-fives, yet, in 1999, ten years after the vaccine had been licensed for use, it was still only available in one low-income country.

The problem was that while vaccinologists and companies want their products to serve everyone, manufacturers initially produced new vaccines at low volume and at such high prices that only wealthier countries could afford their use.[15] The imbalance was striking, and Gro Harlem Brundtland, in a speech to the World Health Assembly, addressed the disequilibrium in quantitative terms that there was a 90/10 problem indelibly associated with the persistence of poverty. 'People in developing countries carry over 90 per cent of the disease burden; yet have access to only 10 per cent of the resources used for health'.[16] Clearly, an impasse existed in the campaign to immunise the world's poorest children. Following the meeting at the World Bank, a small Working Group was formed made up of representatives from WHO, UNICEF, the World Bank, academia and the private sector – their task was to find a way to make new and under-used vaccines more affordable and more accessible to those that needed them the most.

With strong resistance from bilateral agencies opposed to a new structure and with powerful new vaccines against pneumonia and diarrhoea, the two biggest child killers, a new vaccine alliance was desperately required if lives were to be saved. It is always difficult to get groups to work together who cherish their own autonomy, but in March 1984, the Task Force for Child Survival had emerged from a seemingly intractable stalemate. Fifteen years later, in the spring of 1999, the Rockefeller Foundation's Bellagio Centre on Lake Como, one of the great convening locations for the promotion of international understanding, was again the setting for discussions that ultimately led to a fundamental rearrangement of the furniture of global health. Ken Warren, the hyperthymic Director of Health Science at the Rockefeller Foundation, had hosted the 1984 meeting;[17] in 1999, it was the turn of Tim Evans, Director of the Health Equity Theme, of the Rockefeller Foundation to convene a series of meetings at Bellagio aimed at building a successful coalition between competing agencies.

Origins of GAVI

The five meetings held at Bellagio were acrimonious: defined by antagonisms, visceral power plays over operational independence and implacable disagreement between the leading UN agencies: the World Bank, UNICEF and the WHO. Rather than witnessing the emergence of a successful coalition, Tim Evans saw only division.

> The meeting split between the pragmatists and the dreamers. The pragmatists focused on $10 million and a secretariat in Geneva with some private sector engagement. The dreamers believed that we should not be wasting our time here if we are not talking in terms of billions of dollars. The dreamers accused the pragmatists of not having any vision and the pragmatists accused the dreamers of being delusional.[18]

The immunologist, Barry Bloom, was also present during those febrile negotiations and recalls an epiphanic moment when the divide between the factions led to a moment of incredulity.

> I look upon those meetings as one of my most humiliating periods in global health. I was there as an academic without affiliation, and it turned out to be a power struggle between which government agency would succeed the Children's Vaccine Initiative. The arguments between the World Bank, UNICEF and the WHO got so awful, that Herb Pigman,[19] a representative of Rotary International, a farmer from Indiana, looked around the room and asked. 'Why are we here? I thought we were here to save 10 million lives a year with childhood vaccines. How are we going to do that?' I will never forget the poignancy of the moment. He had completely shamed the international organisations. There was dead silence in the room and nothing further to say.[20]

The existing status quo clearly felt vulnerable, with WHO and UNICEF in particular fearing the prospect of a new immunisation partnership that would have its own independent secretariat and revenue stream. They argued that even a small secretariat would grow into a large organization.

The atmosphere of suspicion generated between the partners at Bellagio was an impediment to generating momentum and consensus. Even the reassuring diplomatic skills of Tim Evans had failed to remove the underlying disagreements, this implacable hostility led him to an inevitable conclusion – 'we were stuck'.[21] Clearly, he needed to find someone unperturbed by the size of the challenge, and who possessed the temperament, credibility and management style necessary to operate effectively at the apex of global health decision-making. That was when he decided to phone Tore Godal. Importantly, their professional relationship had begun with an act of thoughtfulness. Early in Tim Evans career, he had applied to TDR for a high-ranking health economist position; Godal then the Director of TDR, 'wrote a personal reply, indicating that while on this occasion, they were looking for someone with more experience, to 'please keep in touch' an encouraging remark, which I've not forgotten'.[22] Some years later, both men worked together on the Multilateral Initiative on Malaria (MIM) a project conceived by the Nobel Prize-winning scientist and Head of the US National Institutes of Health, Harold Varmus, to strengthen research capabilities in malaria endemic countries in Africa. On that occasion, it was Godal in Geneva, who phoned Tim Evans at the Rockefeller Foundation in New York City. He wanted three-quarters of a million dollars to get the MIM up and running. Tim Evans did not take much persuasion; he saw the Multilateral Initiative on Malaria as a very creative model of capacity building, and gave the money to TDR in equal tranches over three years.

> I could make a commitment because I knew Tore was nothing but the best in the business. He did not necessarily have all the good ideas himself, but

he was strategic and shrewd in identifying good ideas and moving them forward. I was relatively new at the Rockefeller that the time, but I felt very secure making that commitment over the phone and then figuring out how to organise it administratively afterwards and getting things through the board of trustees, which would not have been the case if other people had phoned me.[23]

In late April 1999, Evans visited Godal at his home in the village of Morex, close to Geneva, and over breakfast described the leadership problems that were plaguing the Working Group and outlined the potential difficulties that could confront the new alliance when it eventually materialised.[24] However, Tim Evans was confident that whatever complications lay ahead, Godal, as a consummate and trusted global health thinker, would be an effective leader because he practised the quiet, judicious arts necessary to maintain a peaceful coexistence in the tinderbox of a divided community. This inherent skill, honed in the years as Director of TDR, later proved invaluable in enabling an outside agency to help WHO and UNICEF to work together in ways that would have been unthinkable only a few months previously. Indeed, while at TDR Godal's embrace of innovation and close collaborations with large pharmacological companies stood as an exemplar of how the WHO might shed its historic aversion to dealing with the private sector. For many years, Godal, and his TDR colleagues, had worked productively with the eponymous Belgian company Janssen Pharmaceutica in developing drugs against tropical diseases. Godal established a close relationship with Paul Janssen and convinced him that the company should have a public service mission; this enabled TDR to gain access to Janssen's molecule libraries.[25] Moreover, as an immunologist, Godal had a long-standing interest in, and knowledge of, vaccines. Sitting at the breakfast table in Morex, Godal began formulating in his mind the ways in which he could bring focus and leadership to the new alliance; and while the role Evans wanted him to accept lacked formal institutional authority, nevertheless it did offer a tantalising sense of potential. Within the hierarchy of the nascent alliance, there was a Steering Group,[26] advised by the Working Group,[27] made up of a collective of dedicated members spread across institutions in the United States and beyond, acting as the intellectual driver and 'brain trust', interlinked to the leaders of the partner institutions, at the bottom of the governance structure, was the alliance's secretariat. Within weeks, and with the blessing of the Steering Group, Godal simultaneously joined the Working Group and became interim head of the new alliance's secretariat. The design of the administrative architecture appeared at first sight to be deliberately restrictive, devolving little formal power to the head of the secretariat; but Godal, a tactical thinker *par excellence*, identified the existence of an intermediate space within the power dynamic – and his intention was to develop strategies within that intermediate space to modernise global health and transform childhood immunisation.

William Muraskin, in his meticulously researched book, *Crusade to Immunize the World's Children*, wrote very persuasively about the importance of Godal to the new global health alliance,

> The choice of Godal as interim head of the new alliance's secretariat . . . would prove to be one of the most important positive steps taken by the immunization community in increasing the likelihood that the new coalition would survive and prosper.[28]

This opinion from one of the leading researchers of the modern history of immunisation reflects the impact of Godal's contribution to the new endeavour. Experiences gained overseeing previous health care programmes, had taught Godal that the forces of opposition whether internal or external in origin would soon materialise, and while they might be slow off the mark, once marshalled, would be formidable. Hence, the philosophy that underpinned his tenure as executive secretary was, 'momentum, innovation, and look to the future, not the past'.[29] Tireless and single-minded, Godal was determined to move with the times and if this latest attempt to immunise the poorest children was going to succeed then he knew that a new world order in health needed to supplement the existing structure. It was clear to him, and many others in global health, that the WHO, with an annual budget of $1 billion to cover the costs of the entire world's health problems, could not make a significant impact on reducing infectious diseases without collaboration from industry and civil society. There was a need to change the global vaccine landscape and make it work for the people who need it the most. He recognised, and indeed celebrated, the important role played by missionary, Schweitzerian charity-based provision, but with millions of children dying annually from infectious diseases, the business of financing a modern well-resourced programme with supply chains that function properly required serious capacity. Unlike, Halfdan Mahler who created a 'movement' around his vision of 'Health for All by 2000', Godal eschewed the call of an intangible spiritual impulse; in its place he wanted 'to identify something concrete, and then go after it'.[30]

In June 1999, Godal succeeded Tim Evans as the head of the Working Group with a salary paid by the Rockefeller Foundation. To avoid all previous linkages to WHO, his official role was as a consultant to UNICEF, which also parsimoniously supported his appointment with the provision of a secretary, Enyo Asafo, on a part-time basis. It was just as well that Godal did not aspire to a smart suite of offices with a view of the Jet d'Eau in Lake Geneva, because he established the secretariat 'squatting'[31] in a 'dingy dungeon'[32] made up of two offices and a hallway in a former storeroom of UNICEF's basement on Avenue de la Paix. He made the decision for strategic reasons, and on the advice of Gro Harlem Brundtland who wanted the UNICEF locale to prevent any sense of jealousy and fear that WHO would become too strong. GAVI's predecessor, the Children's

Vaccine Initiative (CVI), was hosted but unloved by the WHO, while the outside world saw the CVI as a WHO programme – thereby receiving little insider support and much external suspicion. By physically positioning GAVI in UNICEF's European office, Godal had the benefits of being within the UN system while being free of the New York headquarters' microscopic scrutiny. Besides, Godal was unconcerned about the iconography of workspace surroundings; he was interested in solving problems, which he could do just as effectively from an inauspicious setting as from the elevation of a shiny glass architectural tabernacle, increasingly seen as a necessity for the successful pursuit of knowledge in modern biomedical research. Dating from 1970 and his years as Director of the Armauer Hansen Research Institute in Ethiopia, Godal had grounded experience of doing research in underfunded health systems. This invaluable knowledge prevented him from losing touch with the realities confronting workers in the field. In global health, there is no substitute for feet on the ground, 'mud on boots' fieldwork, and Ethiopia was a life-shaping experience for Godal. Knowing at first hand the effect of the heat, poor roads, poverty, irregular electricity supplies and fractured communication networks enabled him to identify with those desperately trying to provide health care under extremely difficult conditions and to become a more effective public health leader. Immediately upon his appointment, there was a palpable sense of energy, momentum and 'can-do'[33] attitude within the working group. The Executive Director of UNICEF, Carol Bellamy, visited Godal in his so-called dungeon soon after his appointment and recalls the determination that accompanied the austerity.

> Thank goodness for Tore. He was the day-to-day, make-it-happen person. At the secretariat, he had to keep-the-ball-rolling. You knew that if he was involved, there was substance to whatever he was promoting. . . . I remember staring out of his little room, in UNICEF, and him saying, 'we are going to have a lean and keen organisation'. I remember those words, lean and keen, to this very day.[34]

With his title of Executive Secretary, and lodged in UNICEF's Geneva out-post, Godal began making plans to revolutionise the world of immunisation. Although he didn't know it at the time, he was going to be supported in that undertaking by a young US entrepreneurial multibillionaire, turned philanthropist, Bill Gates who also believed in the power of vaccines and the catalytic power of immunisation as an economic development tool.

The First Billion-Dollar Baby

Bill Gates is the modern-day equivalent of the legendary US business magnate John D. Rockefeller. Like his predecessor, the generosity of his benefactions to medical research helped to transform the health and well-being of millions of people. At the end of the nineteenth century, the Baptist clergyman, and thinker Frederick Taylor Gates, persuaded Rockefeller that his accumulated fortune would achieve the greatest utility if invested in advancing medical science, modernizing medical education and finding cures for debilitating parasitic diseases like hookworm that caused poverty and held back national efficiency. One hundred years later, in 1997, Bill Gates after visiting India and witnessing the suffering caused by polio and other preventable diseases, asked Bill Foege, a former director of the US Centers for Disease Control and Prevention, how he could learn and contribute to the field of global health.[35] Foege gave the 41-year-old billionaire a reading list of 82 books. One of those on the reading list was the World Bank's *World Development Report 1993: Investing in Health.* Gates found the study so utterly persuasive that he 'read it twice'.[36] The logic of the statistical analysis showing how good health increases the economic productivity of individuals and the economic growth rates of countries, convinced Gates that investing in health would be a cost-effective use of his fortune. Bill Gates Jr. had built his computer company, Microsoft, on the meticulous analysis of numerical data as a way of making value free, metric-driven decisions. *Investing in Health* showed Gates that good health for everyone in the world, even the poorest, was attainable through the targeted use of vaccines, primary health care programmes, diagnostics and drugs. Gates, like others before him, saw the persuasive logic of the Harvard microbiologist Geoffrey Edsall's classical statement made in 1963, that 'never in the history of human progress has a better and cheaper method of preventing illness been developed than immunization at its best'.[37] The sole requirement was an institution, or an individual with the vision, leadership and financial power to make it happen. However, even Gates was not wealthy enough to make everyone in the world rich; but if the right programmes against the most harmful preventable diseases were determined by an entrepreneurial metric-driven philanthropy, there was an opportunity to close the health gap between the poorest and richest members of the global community. Increasingly in global health thinking, *health* is *wealth*.[38] James Wolfensohn, the then president of the World Bank, having travelled widely in developing countries was passionate about global inequalities, and wanted the bank to be 'more efficient and effective in . . . reducing poverty'.[39] Importantly, as a Gates business model, there was a synergy between software development and vaccines, in that both were complex and expensive to develop, but comparatively easy to apply.

Initially called the William H. Gates Foundation, in the early days the young Bill Gates entrusted the dispensing of funds to his father, Bill Gates, Sr., who had one assistant, Suzanne Cluett. Far from being prototypical of the mega-philanthropy of later years, this was in the words of Tim Evans, 'kitchen table philanthropy',[40] and the first check written was for $80,000 donated to a local cancer program. Gradually, the combination of the meticulous calculation of numerical data allied to expert advice from global health luminaries like the Australian immunologist, Sir Gus Nossal,[41] and the Canadian physician,

Gordon Perkin a co-founder of PATH,[42] expanded the philanthropic sphere of activity geographically and in terms of health objectives. Gordon Perkin became a trusted advisor of the elder Gates, and in the final months of 1998, PATH launched the Children's Vaccine Program (CVP) with a donation of $100 million from the Gates family. Mark Kane, a long-time WHO employee (seconded from the CDC in Atlanta) and member of the Bellagio Working Group, led the Children's Vaccine Program. By way of a conciliatory gesture, before the failed Bellagio meetings ended in disarray, Mark Kane invited all of the participants to meet again in Seattle in mid-July 1999, to design a programme of immunization for the twenty-first century. As the date came closer, Godal had only a matter of weeks to prepare for the all-important meeting at the Gates Foundation in Seattle.

The Working Group reconvened in offices on the waterfront in Seattle under Godal's leadership and rapidly developed a new vaccine programme that would strengthen routine immunisation and introduce underutilised vaccines. Over two days, with Barry Bloom acting as chair, the structure of the new initiative including the board, and the secretariat, began to take shape. On the eve of the meeting with the Gates delegation, the only thing missing was a name for their new commitment. The room divided over the choice of keeping the Children's Vaccines Initiative, or the entirely new taxonomy of the Global Partnership for Vaccines and Immunization (GPVI). Bloom favouring the linguist allusion of 'alliance' over 'partnership' used his vote to break the tie and the Global Alliance for Vaccines and Immunization (GAVI) formally came into existence. If the new alliance was going to succeed in achieving its audacious aims to make new and under-used vaccines more affordable and more accessible to those that needed them the most, a very large benefaction was going to be required.

The meeting took place on 12–13 July 1999, chaired by Bill Gates Sr., and at his side sat Patty Stonesifer, a former Microsoft senior executive and now CEO of the Bill and Melinda Gates Foundation. The representatives of the WHO, UNICEF, World Bank and industry all sang from same hymn sheet and presented a united front because they knew that if the belligerence of Bellagio resurfaced in Seattle, then no new money would be forthcoming. Moreover, support would be conditional and undergirded by a philosophy that demanded a performance-based system that was cost-effective, time limited and with a more entrepreneurial focus than the traditional overseas development programmes that went on underfunded in perpetuity. At one stage, there was a discussion about research funds for new vaccines, and Bill Gates Sr., replied, 'Research, it is a bottomless pit. We can't get into that'.[43] More worryingly, Bill Gates Sr. told the meeting that the foundation 'would not invest in agencies like WHO and UNICEF',[44] and for a moment Godal thought that embargo would also apply to GAVI. On this occasion, his anxiety was misplaced; at the end of the meeting Godal, the de facto leader of the GAVI, and others met with Bill Sr. and Patty Stonesifer, and were invited to develop a proposal of not more than five pages in length, for Bill Jr., to read. The requested brevity made it possible for the multibillionaire – still fully occupied being CEO and Chairman of the board of Microsoft – to scrutinise the proposal while on the golf course. The application carried one further restriction: it could not exceed $750 million! The stakes were high, and no wonder Godal felt 'star struck'[45] at the thought of securing such an unprecedented sum to translate intensions into action. The next day, the GAVI delegation wrote the five-page proposal in the offices of PATH and submitted it for review.

The conference of the so-called Proto-Board in Seattle forms a key event in the long history of immunisation; in addition to successfully controlling the undercurrents of distrust between the agencies, it also allowed the Gates Foundation to see at first-hand the calibre of the GAVI personnel. Importantly, the foundation got a measure of Godal as a negotiator and his diplomatic approach that favoured pragmatism over ideological purity and compromise over confrontation, which held out the promise that people could work together with common purpose. Of course, it undoubtedly helped that Bill Foege had been an admirer and friendly ally of Godal, 'for as long as I can remember', not only that Foege had been classmates with Gro Harlem Brundtland in 1965 when they studied for a Master of Public Health (MPH) degree at Harvard. Although Godal was notoriously laconic – 'deeds not words' is the mantra – those who worked with him were sure of one thing; that he could be trusted and that he would never say things that he did not mean. Never.[46] Within less than a month, the logic of the transformational roadmap outlined in the five-page proposal, combined with Godal's monogamous commitment to the programme of transforming immunisation coverage, persuaded Bill Gates Jr., to donate $750 million to GAVI over five years. At the time, Bill Gates Jr. was the richest person in the world, but even for him, the unparalleled size the donation caused visible anxiety, and when he signed the cheque, he remembers that his hand was shaking.[47]

Godal knew that if GAVI was going to successfully transform the global inoculation landscape, it would need to make the unique public–private business model work, be innovative, courageous, and most importantly of all, focus on speed of delivery. In the days that followed, his laser-like focus on bringing powerful new vaccine technology to those who needed it most was echoed by a philosophical principle he had defined just three years earlier. 'The challenge to those who wish to use science for a purpose is a challenge of pragmatic opportunism: we must keep in touch with and leap at every chance and make of it as best we can'.[48] He was not alone in giving his best; in terms of dedication, sheer intellectual horsepower and relentless creativity, the Working Group was indispensable to Godal's survival and that of the fledgling alliance. The donation was a leap of faith by the Gates Foundation and the leadership and money that flowed into GAVI over the next five years transformed global health thinking. Gus Nossal is one of the world's leading vaccine researchers and was an advisor to the Gates Foundation in the early days when it was looking for ways to make a lasting impact on global health.

> I think the Gates Foundation was pivotal in two ways. Firstly, the largesse of the contribution, speaking about billions for the first time and not millions. Secondly, it was the importance of the symbolism – that one of the world's richest people would come in, under the banner of global health, put his prestige on the line, and urge others to join him creating a wide philanthropic movement, not just leaving the job to governments that had been the case before. That is very, very important.[49]

There is little doubt that since Edward Jenner's introduction of a smallpox vaccine over 200 years ago the lines of the history and the ideals of global health converge in individual lives. Possibly, it was only those Bellagio 'dreamers' of a new healthcare era and, who rejected the failings of the status quo, could have imagined such a game-changing investment, and one that served as a precursor of the growing power of private capital in the politics of global health.

Tore Godal: The Glue That Hold Things Together

In his role as an international public servant, Godal wanted the new programme of childhood vaccinations to change the world. In the weeks leading up to the first Board Meeting of GAVI, held at UNICEF House in New York on 28 October 1999, increasingly he found powerful allies within the Norwegian state. In fact, it is impossible to separate Godal's Norwegian heritage and his work in global health, from the moral, economic and political support that he could call upon. In the country's modern history, Norway had a world-renowned proficiency in the areas of conflict resolution, development, environmentalism and gender equality, but not in the field of health. At the end of 1990s, across the political spectrum in Norway, this relatively new adherence to global health engagement created a sense of national pride when Gro Harlem Brundtland became the Director-General of the WHO, and simultaneously the first Chair of GAVI. In the decade either side of the new millennium, a growing belief in global health united the nation around socially conscious policies, a feature exemplified by the Norwegian Ministry of Health actively pursuing a policy of international solidarity believing that the best way to protect the well-being of the Norwegian people was to invest in global health. This recalibration of political mores presented Godal with an opportunity to orchestrate a consensus within the wider political culture that subordinated national self-interest to the *love-thy-neighbour* traditions of Norway's Christian missionary movement, and the ethos of solidarity and *help-those-who-are-in-need* beliefs of the nation's Labour movement. Pragmatic opportunism once more offered him the convening power to push global health up the political agenda and form a bridge seamlessly linking domestic politics to Norad, the Norwegian overseas development aid agency. Importantly, Norway did not have an imperial past unlike many of the other countries that pioneered tropical medical research. This cultural legacy further confirmed Godal's suitability as the leader of GAVI, a health programme that linked the developed northern economies and countries in the Global South.

At the policy level, the driving force in the development of GAVI continued to be the Working Group composed of Amie Batson (World Bank), Steve Landry (USAID), Violaine Mitchell (Task Force on Finance), Mike Levine (University of Maryland), Mark Kane (BMGF), Jaques Francois Martin (Vaccine Industry), Suomi Sakai (UNICEF), Michel Zaffran (WHO) and with Godal as chair. This small group had been working closely together for some months, forming bonds of friendship and finding inventive technical solutions to vaccination bottlenecks, before Godal succeeded Tim Evans as their leader. According to Amie Batson, 'we were all die-hard committed'[50] to GAVI's mission to promote the right of every child to be protected against vaccine-preventable diseases. 'So, when Tore came in, we were all [of the mind-set that] 'the jury's still out' . . . a feeling of 'let's wait and see' healthy scepticism'.[51] These feelings of uncertainty were soon replaced by a sense of respect, as the Working Group were won over by Godal's lack of ego, and refusal to waiver in his ambition to do what some believed was impossible; end the time delay between the introduction of new vaccines in rich countries and their use in the poorest regions of the world. The Working Group was in the main a virtual entity, as it was spread geographically across the United States and Europe, with each of the individual members working from the offices of their home institutions in Geneva, New York City, Seattle or Washington, DC. The cultural integrity and levels of ambition of the group being fostered through weekly conference calls, where ideas were fine-tuned and proposals rigorously interrogated. Face-to-face quarterly meetings, which rotated in succession among the partner organisations, strengthened lines of communications further and collectively designed GAVI's strategic way forward. Godal's commitment to do what was right for the wider community rather than enhance his own power and kudos received widespread recognition in the early history of GAVI. In December 1999, Jeff Sachs, chair of the WHO Commission on Macroeconomics and Health, invited Godal to co-chair a panel with him on R&D. Sachs looked upon Godal as, 'an inspiration, guru and teacher'[52] and someone capable of finding technical solutions and political support for public health programmes. One month later, when the Working Group met on the eve of the official launch of GAVI, on 23 January, at the World Economic Forum, in Davos, Godal relayed Sachs's offer to his colleagues. No one thought that it was a good idea, and Amie Batson expressed grave and explicit concerns.

We all said, 'this is a total conflict of interest, you cannot do that' and Godal reflected for a moment, and agreed saying, 'yes, you're right. I need to fully focus on GAVI'. I remember thinking this is the measure of Tore. He listens and he does what is right. This is a leader that I can follow.[53]

There are many components to building a relationship based on trust, and on that day high in the Rhaetian Alps of Switzerland, Godal won the trust of the Working Group with an act of selflessness.

In the lifecycle of any new global organisation, the most difficult period is the early start-up phase of getting governance established and the systems up and running. Initially, the plan was for GAVI to exist for only five years, and with a budget of $750 million, Godal's primary objective was to bring vaccine technology to those who needed it most, the children in the world's poorest 75 countries. The day-to-day running of the health programme would fall to the Secretariat. In order for GAVI to succeed, and avoid the pitfalls of past vaccination programmes, Godal knew that he would need to take drastic action to get things done quickly, even if that meant discarding conventional rules, management structures and bureaucratic allegiances. He also knew that his approach

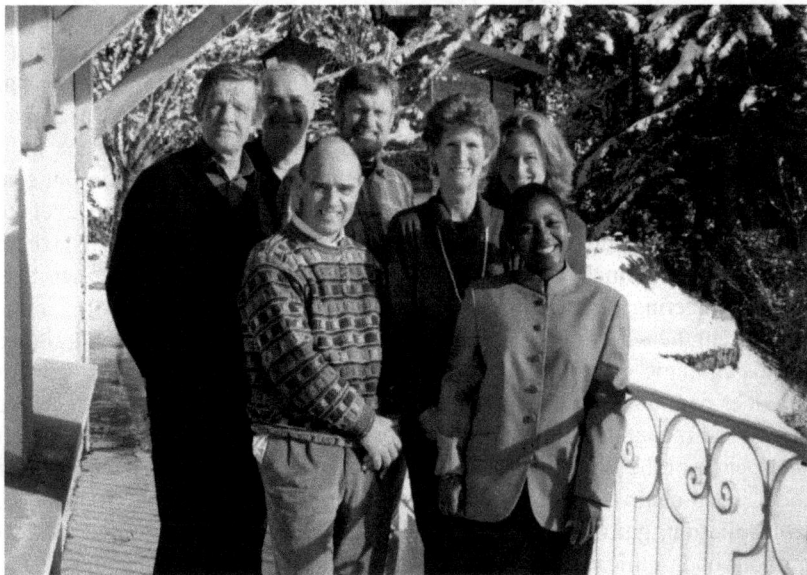

Figure 4.1 An example of Tore Godal's lean and light-touch management style was reflected in the GAVI Secretariat holding a work meeting at a restaurant in the Jura Mountains above Geneva, January 2001. It was their first ever office planning retreat. After finishing work, the team went cross-country skiing. Left to right, Tore Godal, Umberto Cancellieri, Ivone Rizzo, Bo Stenson, Jane Dryhauge, Lisa Jacobs, Enyonam Asafo.

Source: Courtesy of Bo Stenson.

would be tendentious, but he was determined to do whatever was required to make GAVI's unique public–private business model succeed, and if this led to him losing his job, 'then so be it'.[54] In 1986, when Godal visited the American epidemiologist D. A. Henderson, who had directed the international effort to eradicate smallpox 20 years before, his advice was 'break all the rules, but keep on good terms with Finance and Personnel'. Those two elements, *money* and *people*, moulded the arc of GAVI's contribution to the history of global health. Bill Gates Sr. travelled to Geneva in the early days of the venture where Godal showed his distinguished visitor around the two-room GAVI headquarters. Both men shared an operational ideal, 'do things in a simple way, and don't waste money'. In these face-to-face talks, it was decided that GAVI would receive an annual instalment of $150 million over five years. Now with funding assured, Godal began recruiting the Secretariat whose job it would be to dispense the vaccine programme to its intended beneficiaries.

The secretariat grew slowly, because while speed was of the essence, Godal wanted to make sure that he recruited people who were competent and dedicated to seizing the opportunity to change the architecture of global health. Initially, he hired staff on a consultancy basis to test them out before appointing them on formal contracts. From the outset, his aim was to recruit a small number of good people that would take ownership of the programme; experience had taught him that the more people there are the greater the propensity for waste, replication and omission. The first person recruited was Bo Stenson, a Swedish health systems specialist who had been responsible for WHO matters at the Swedish International Development Cooperation Agency (SIDA). Bo had known Godal since the TDR days of the late 1970s. He was a good manager, a clear thinker, and had a deep understanding of the politics of world health. The next recruit was Ivone Rizzo, a quiet Italian, seconded from UNICEF, who was a terrific number cruncher. In contrast, Godal then appointed Lisa Jacobs, a dynamic American with a background in journalism who was able to write reports quickly, and being an excellent networker, established seamless lines of communication linking the Secretariat with the other GAVI bodies. The final member of the group was Umberto Cancellieri, a manager with a background in operations and responsible for finance in the UNICEF office in Geneva. Because of his UNICEF background, Cancellieri was well connected across global health agencies, and his warm and welcoming personality helped to get people on side.

From the outset, Godal's management style was 'light touch' giving his team the freedom and responsibility to build GAVI into an alliance with the deliberate intention of making the WHO, UNICEF, the Gates Foundation and others feel that *they* were in charge, and that the Secretariat was their servant.[55] His objective was to make the members play the central role and feel that they did so. This was a strategic decision, because if disagreements did surface between agencies, the deferentially aligned secretariat would occupy the position of trusted arbitrator, and not appear as a separate powerbroker. Godal reinforced this sentiment through his own actions, which unambiguously merged public service and anonymity. He kept a conspicuously low profile in public, intentionally putting himself on the back row in group photographs, preferring to concentrate his attentions on the political battles and scientific disagreements that he knew lay ahead. Godal's foremost quality as a leader according to Bo Stenson, was his political astuteness.

> I think this was part of his genius. Tore's real interests were in the political aspects, the strategic aspects of seeing 'how could you handle the members? What were their interests? And finding ways to make them work together without getting stuck in conflicts'.[56]

In this way, Godal was able to evade the mistrust and bureaucratic jealousies that had undermined GAVI's predecessor, the Children's Vaccine Initiative.

The secretariat, selected by Godal for their complementary skills, was in no doubt that their boss had set his life on making GAVI a success. An idealist with an eye for practical reform, he was determined to stop the immunisation failures of the past resurfacing in the present. 'One of the things I still remember from working with Tore twenty-years ago', recalls Lisa Jacobs, who was in charge of communications and governance,

> is make a reasonable timetable and stick to it. It is such an easy win to make a promise and keep to it. Because the UN was terrible about setting unrealistic deadlines, that they would never meet and [therefore] no one expects them to meet. When we set deadlines, we met them. That is very important to him.[57]

Few people who were not members of the organisations in which Godal worked can have any appreciation of the contribution he made to global health, because he was devoid of personal ambition, except for the welfare of the bodies, which he served. In order to understand how he persuaded people, by example, to work together to improve the health of the planet, we need to understand more about how he saw the world, how he interacted with others, and the enigmatic nature of his character. Once Godal had assembled his small team to run the programmatic and technical side of GAVI's operations, every day began in the same way. 'We were all in one big room, Tore had his room off to the side', Lisa Jacobs recounts,

> and about 0930 or so, he would emerge from his office and always used the same phrase: 'So, how about a coffee?' We would all then go up to the eighth floor where UNICEF had its canteen, and we had coffee and lunch together every day – we didn't have any formal meetings.[58]

Bo Stenson calculated that over the five years of Godal's leadership thousands of these working breaks took place which in addition to establishing smooth

coordination within the office fostered a sense of camaraderie. 'I liked the atmosphere which was great from the start. We were a small closely-knit group with a
commitment and loyalty to Tore. He trusted us, and always asked "what would
you like to do now?"'[59] Godal's light-touch management style, and quiet confidence transfused through the team and by way of osmotic understanding helped
to create a shared dedication to make GAVI a sustainable model of global health
for the twenty-first century. To succeed where others had failed, Godal knew that
in order to put GAVI on the map as a public–private organisation, it had to have
a very strong balance sheet and a very credible way to buy vaccines.

Money and Politics

Many expected that the launch of the GAVI in Davos would mobilise international philanthropy and corporations with eleemosynary leanings to contribute
to immunising the world's children, but no organisation pledged additional funding. Even a special fundraising meeting held in the White House, chaired by
President Bill Clinton in the final days of his administration, failed to persuade
the representatives of the pharmaceutical companies of the righteousness of the
cause. Standing near the back of the cabinet room, the tall Norwegian attempted
to leaven the despondency. 'I'm the only person in this room that will be fired if
the programme fails'. Looking at Godal, President Clinton replied, 'Don't worry,
and blame it on me. I will soon be out of office'.[60] Godal knew that Bill Gates
and his staff were becoming increasingly anxious that other funders were not
coming forward, and behind the scenes, he kept pushing decision-makers to join
a project that was the most efficient and cost-effective way to protect vulnerable
life. A decisive moment in the history of global immunization occurred in March
2000 when the leader of the Norwegian Labour Party, Jens Stoltenberg, became
Prime Minister of Norway. Godal was eager to meet the new prime minister
and through the combined efforts of Gro Harlem Brundtland and Jonas Gahr
Støre, Stoltenberg's Chief of Staff, the two men met for the first time. One of
Godal's exceptional abilities is to reach that level in the listener's mind at which
the spark of recognition jumps the gap and ignites understanding. This was just
such an occasion. 'Tore is a softly spoken person, with a very strong and clear
message', Jens Stoltenberg recalled, 'and he convinced me that I should make
vaccines and immunisation a big project for my new government'.[61] As a trained
economist and statistician, the cost-effectiveness of vaccines, with their compelling amalgamation of low cost for huge effect' was intellectually and politically
attractive to Stoltenberg. As an indication of his government's solidarity with the
ideal of inoculating the world's children, Stoltenberg invited the GAVI Board
to hold their spring meeting at the Holmenkollen Park Hotel in Oslo, Norway.
In his opening speech, Stoltenberg announced in almost apologetic terms[62] that
he would donate one billion kroner (close to US$150 million) over five years to
GAVI. The declaration caused a great outpouring of emotion, particularly from

Bill Gates Sr. who saw Norway's generous allocation of state funds not only as a vindication of his son's vision for improving global health but also as a harbinger of additional monies to come. Godal confessed that he was 'overwhelmed' by his compatriot's generosity, and later at the meeting in Oslo, the Dutch development minister, Everline Herfkens emboldened by Norway's benefaction, confirmed that her government would match the Norwegian contribution. Other countries, including the United Kingdom soon followed Norway's lead in giving long-term financial commitments, which enabled GAVI to become the first public–private 'billion-dollar baby' in the history of global health. The early conversion of Jens Stoltenberg to the cause of 'Vaccination Against Poverty' had a profound impact on Norwegian politics, the life scientific of Godal, and the health of millions of women and children in low- and middle-income countries in the first quarter of the twenty-first century. In this way, Stoltenberg forms part of a philosophical continuum in the post-war history of Norway, like Gro Harlem Brundtland, Jonas Gahr Støre,[63] Anniken Huitfeldts and indeed his own sister, the public health academic and activist, Camilla Stoltenberg – he was a strong supporter of development aid. Instinctively, he knew that it was important to help people, but the great conundrum was – what were the moral obligations of development assistance? How could he unite Norway's Christian socialist philanthropy to the ethical underpinnings of global health and development?[64] To maintain the public's confidence, he was determined to spend the big money on the big issues, and one of those was what he described as the vaccine miracle.[65] 'The beauty of the GAVI', in Stoltenberg's rational mind,

> is that immunisation is the best way to fight poverty and you could measure the impact. That was the message from Tore, and it was the reason why Norway was the first nation to join GAVI. The Gates Foundation were pleased, because while they have a lot of financial strength, they felt it was important to team up with others.[66]

The fortuitous amalgamation of the public and private sectors was a GAVI innovation and a model that later became commonplace in other sectors of development outside health. The Gates Foundation, whose visionary philanthropy embodies a business-like utilitarianism, moved into a more public-sector sphere, an area traditionally dominated by public-facing agencies and governments. Thus, GAVI was a merger of the best elements of the entrepreneurial approach that Bill and Melinda Gates and Patty Stonesifer thought necessary, intertwined with the long-term view of making improved global health central to a country's foreign policy, and one that looked beyond the Wall Street timescale of 'the next quarter' or 'the next year'. This was the successful model that propelled GAVI forward, and which critically had eluded previous attempts to inoculate the world's poorest children.

The Dynamic First Years of GAVI

The first principle of GAVI was speed. Guided by Godal's strategic insight, the team decided to focus on countries with a GDP per capita of less than US$1,000. However, that included three countries with very large populations: China, India and Indonesia.[67] In order to keep within budgetary constraints, GAVI had to adopt special allocations for them. 'There we faced another challenge, vaccine prices', remembered Godal almost two decades later.

> We had a heated discussion within the WG on this and Jacques-Francois argued in favoured of a differentiated price, i.e. the lowest price for the poorest countries, and the highest for high income countries. Others contended that we should have a flat price for everyone. In the end, I was asked to suggest a differentiated price for Gro, The chair of the interim Board. I was very anxious when I asked her, as I thought she would say no. But, to my surprise she said yes, so that became the decision.[68]

All together 75 countries became eligible, with a child cohort of about 90 million out of 130 million globally. 'Simplicity was an important principle' recalled Godal, 'so we decided on a programme in which children would receive three doses of diphtheria-tetanus-pertussis (DPT3) and in due course that would also include Hep B and Hib'.[69] Godal, an idealist with an eye for practical reform, wanted to introduce an element of competition in the form of results-based financing, with financial incentives paid for every extra child vaccinated. For GAVI to be successful, there needed to be evidence that vaccination strategies had the full commitment of their governments, and that they would save lives. When the application process was being discussed within the Working Group, Amie Batson suggested that to avoid any suggestion of partisanship, applications should be reviewed by an independent expert committee, which would have the advantage of depoliticizing the selection process and bring a greater sense of fairness. This suggestion had an immediate appeal to Godal, because when he had been the Head of TDR, an independent body of scientists reviewed all funding applications. The inherent attraction of replicating this system of impartial adjudication ensured its immediate incorporation into the programmatic design. Godal was also keen that the composition of the proposed Independent Review Committee should have a majority of health scientists from the Global South. Under the leadership of the Thai public health physician Viroj Tangcharoensathien, the Independent Review Committee (IRC) became an enlightened invention, acting as a firewall against external political pressures from recalcitrant governments, and as arbiter in any internal machinations brought by members of the GAVI board or other powerful elements. By the early summer of 2000, the frantic pace being set bought the first large tranche of country applications to the office of the Secretariat in Geneva. Viroj Tangcharoensathien was conscientious and experienced; he had been an active member of the Scientific and Technical Advisory Committee of TDR in the early 1990s, and he was not going to merely rubber stamp country applications without proper consideration.

> When I was first asked to lead the IRC, I felt hesitant, but when I realised that GAVI was such an innovative programme in global health, I said yes. My job was to develop a system of assessment and evaluation. When we had a dispute, I thought that Tore was over influenced by the narrow view of the magic bullet of vaccines, whereas I thought we also needed strong health systems, otherwise it becomes a series of silos. . . . GAVI saved a huge number of lives in China by making an impact on the prevalence of hepatitis, and vaccine coverage globally increased greatly. The Secretariat was only five people managing a $750 million budget. They really had to work.[70]

An inimitable feature of GAVI is its co-financing model. All governments, no matter how poor, contribute towards the cost of every vaccine they receive. This contribution increases as the wealth of the country increases, until the time arrives when the recipient country pays the total cost of the vaccine. This innovation had the effect of cajoling and at the same time, rewarding governments to assign funds for inoculation programmes that would promote the health of children under the age of 5. By this mechanism, GAVI succeeded in bringing to the fore one of the guiding principles of the 1946 Constitution of the World Health Organization: 'Governments have a responsibility for the health of their peoples'. This was the long-term vision of health care that Godal wanted to disseminate as a means of reducing the burden of disease. Not having vaccine programmes eternally dependent on foreign aid programmes is one of the most important durable and deliberate features of GAVI. Alice Albright was GAVI's Chief Financial Officer for the first nine years of its existence.

> We took the view that GAVI should not be a permanent subsidizer of vaccines such that it would displace governments' ultimate responsibility. It pushed children higher up the political agenda and suddenly under-five mortality is something that gets money behind it – as it should. And this century there has been a phenomenal 50% reduction in under-five mortality. This has never happened before. GAVI, Tore and others deserve our gratitude for that.[71]

Within 20 years of GAVI's inception, a transformation had taken place in global health with more than 85% of children vaccinated against diphtheria, tetanus and pertussis, and 90% receiving at least one vaccine. Winston Churchill once admiringly said of his political opponent, Joseph Chamberlain that he 'made the weather', meaning that he set the agenda for other politicians to follow. To adapt Churchill's phrase, GAVI under Godal's prescient political skills made the weather in terms of global health governance at the beginning of a new millennium.

Solving Historic Problems

To avoid past failures and speed up the progress of universal childhood immunization, Godal displayed a wanton disregard for rules and management structure.[72]
Results were what he cared about most and he was prepared to do whatever it
took to get them. He was constantly scanning the horizon for ideas; the hallmarks
of his tenure were elevating the level of ambition and to inspire people to change
the world. Dominating all was the concept of speed, and only two-and-a-half
years after GAVI's launch, the Independent Review Committee had approved
36 countries for support. Such rapid progress was possible because of the common thread of trust that existed between the countries and GAVI, and between
Godal and his colleagues. Also, by working directly with Ministers of Health,
Godal was able to circumvent the sclerotic effect of WHO Regional Offices, a
process designed to expedite the application process. Of course, the path was not
always smooth. Godal was driven by an ethical compunction to maintain children's immunisation as a central policy objective for the world community; he
also wanted to immunise millions of children throughout the developing world
against hepatitis B, and all this had to be achieved within a five-year timeframe.
With so much to do and time in such short supply, it is not surprising that Godal's
forward-leaning vision for inoculation and desire for bold action meant that in
terms of policy and objectives, he occasionally found himself precariously far
out in front of the status quo. In March 2000, the Norwegian physician Paul Fife
succeeded Suomi Sakai as the UNICEF representative on the Working Group;
from this vantage point, he was able to offer an insight into his compatriot's
modus operandi.

> Trying to keep up with Tore is like chasing a downhill skier who has no regard
> for the boulders. At his peak, he was very physical and amazing at moving
> things forward. You would have a conversation with him, and a day later, he
> was on the other side of the world having conversations with politicians. He is
> very much a people person and that is very much a Norwegian trait.[73]

All the members of the Working Group could see that Godal's objective was not
personal advancement,[74] and while acknowledging that he had an uncanny apti-
tude for choosing winning policies, he did, on occasion hit a metaphorical boul-
der. When his colleagues felt that by accelerating ahead, he was going beyond
the consensus, or that his unwavering campaigns to persuade ministers of health
to deliver immunisation services were taking him away from Geneva for too
long, then they would attempt to reel in his enthusiasms. Just such a moment
occurred when the Working Group launched a new financial programme that
required complex sequential decisions to be made in order to translate intensions
into action; however, progress was not being made fast enough for Godal and
he decided to hit the campaign trail in order to shake things up. This did not go

down well with Violaine Mitchell who was coordinating the rollout of the programme and she decided to take an unconventional approach.

> Tore had an incredible network of ministers and deputy ministers of health that he had built up during his TDR days, and he would grab the famous little overnight bag he kept in his office and fly off. At the time, I had a sheep farm, and I had one particularly difficult sheep that was constantly getting stuck in fences, and going off by itself, so I bought it a horrible bell. And so, for Christmas that year, I grabbed the bell off the sheep, wrapped it in some wool, and sent it to Tore with a note which read, 'Please wear this and just let us know where you are!'[75]

Aberrational behaviour aside, one of Godal's signal accomplishments was to build a positively reinforcing cycle that succeeded in persuading all the partners to understand that there was a greater good above that of their own institution or their own perspective. Moreover, that by contributing to the selflessness of the alliance they would also better serve their own objectives. By harnessing this ethos of collective responsibility, Amie Batson sensed that times were changing in global health, 'this was going into a new world order, where health is not just the purview of WHO, it is the purview of all of the partners'.[76] Through some extraordinary process of subliminal engagement, Godal created a culture based on his principled leadership that shaped the philosophy of the organisation. In fact, this shared adhesion to the moral and medical values of the alliance was so strong; Godal later noted that, 'members of the Working Group over time became more loyal to GAVI than to their home institutions'.[77]

In the modern history of medicine, key discoveries like those of penicillin, ivermectin and chlorpromazine have contributed to the upward arc of human health, and so too have the impact of new fields of research including cancer epidemiology, genetics and molecular biology. Some of these improvements came about through serendipity, or rational drug design, while others were the culmination of the slow accretion of scientific knowledge over time. Rarely, in the modern world have profound scientific advances been made by individuals in the manner of Edward Jenner, Paul Ehrlich or Dorothy Hodgkin. However, we should not overlook the significance of individual agency in the history of global health; and it would be a distortion of history to underestimate the impact of Bill Foege and DA Henderson in the eradication of smallpox, or the persuasive power of Richard Doll's medical statistical studies in transforming our understanding of the dangers of smoking. Likewise, in making an attempt to analyse Godal's contribution to global health – bearing in mind that some see his legacy as being public service and anonymity – at times we need to understand his role as a scientist, together with his mastery of being an international public servant. Some of these skills are tangible and comprehensible relating to day-to-day administrative guile, while others are hard to define and transcendental. To Bill Foege, it was, 'being able to make people work together', while Violaine Mitchell saw it as being able to 'make the impossible possible'; to Lisa Jacobs, 'he was so inscrutable, people would listen to him, there was something special, he is not like us, he is some kind of deity'; Amie Batson saw him as, 'a force of nature, very strategic, and once he has made up his mind, he is not afraid of failing. I think he is the best leader I have ever worked with'; in the eyes of Alice Albright, 'there is this quiet confidence and stubbornness in the best sense of the word. I was lucky to work for him and I would do it again in two seconds'; for Paul Fife there was also something that was unquantifiable,

> He is good with complex matters, with timing and the ability to always be there at the right moment. It talks of Tore's magic, because he's not a very charismatic person, he is amazing at moving issues forward, but the point is to understand it you need to be there with him.

Vaccines Do Not Save Lives. Vaccinations Save Lives

The secret of GAVI's success was its unique public–private business model, in conjunction with the innovative way that it raised funds for childhood vaccinations. The great financial leap forward was the creation of the International Finance Facility for Immunisation, or IFFIm, which was the brainchild of Gordon Brown, the UK Chancellor of the Exchequer (Finance Minister) in Tony Blair's Labour government. Brown shared a background of Christian socialist philanthropy with his close ally on global health and development, Norway's Prime Minister Jens Stoltenberg. As a politician, Brown was devoted to reducing poverty at home and abroad and to finding inventive ways to put development on the map. In 2020, Brown recalled the genealogy of the concept, 'IFFIm was an idea I worked on with Baroness Shriti Vadera, we believed we could generate substantial money for GAVI. I presented at its launch, and Norway, Italy and France and other countries joined'.[78] The idea underpinning IFFIm is to mobilise large sums on money quickly by using long-term pledges from donor governments to sell bonds in capital markets, making funds immediately available for GAVI programmes. The borrowing being backed by legally binding pledges from governments to reimburse investors from future aid budgets. The mechanism is analogous to buying a house with a mortgage and designed to channel more aid to developing countries. In November 2003, Alice Albright and her financial team began working on the details of the mechanism: 'IFFIm gave GAVI the financial teeth to compete in the vaccine market, and not just to be noticed: but to drive the price of vaccines down and to make a commitment to buy ahead'.[79] Since 2006, IFFIm has raised US$6.5 billion towards a range of programmes, from health system strengthening to emergency vaccine stockpiles. The success of this financial mechanism, a product of the close collaboration between Brown and Stoltenberg, led to a breakthrough in generosity as well as science. Paralleling the scientific expertise inside government, new economic theories were being developed to help improve people's lives. Invented and championed by the US economist Michael Kremer[80] was the Advanced Market Commitment (AMC), which changed the way GAVI and the vaccine-producing companies worked together. The AMC addressed the research and development problems within the pharmaceutical companies and the imbalance that led to 90% of the R&D budget targeting only 10% of the diseases affecting the global community. The AMC spoke to this market failure and enabled GAVI, according to Alice Albright, to say to the powerful vaccine-producing companies.

> If you finish the research and development on your rotavirus vaccine we will *guarantee* to pay you at a level that creates an incentive for you to finish the R&D process quickly, so that we can vaccinate children against severe diarrhoea, a leading cause of disease in low income countries.[81]

Through this groundbreaking policy, GAVI enabled R&D programmes to be fast-tracked that might otherwise have been considered financially unattractive to finish. One of the most important allowed manufacturers to speed up production and distribution of the Pneumococcal vaccine for more than 140 million children in 56 different countries in just six years.[82] The clarity of the cost-effectiveness of the financing vehicle became apparent when Godal was involved in negotiating a price for Pneumococcal vaccine of US$3.50 per dose on the Advanced Market Commitment, down from US$48.00 in the United States. Thus, through a combination of political leadership and strategic engagement, the market failures that had plagued previous attempts by the international community to find cost-effective treatments for deadly childhood diseases were disappearing. GAVI pooled demand from developing countries and guaranteed manufacturers long-term, high-volume and predictable markets; in return, vaccine manufacturers increased their production and reduced their prices to levels that low-income countries could afford.

Developing a vaccine is an immense achievement, and so too is distributing it; ultimately all vaccination campaigns are dependent upon the availability of vaccines. Of course, vaccines do not deliver themselves and consequently health system strengthening has been at the core of GAVI's work from the very beginning, accounting for about 25% of total investments. In part, as a response to the campaigning zeal of people like Bo Stenson and Viroj Tangcharoensathien, for long-term investments in health systems and capacity building to ensure inoculations are successfully delivered in poor countries. In growing the size of the economic pie, GAVI also improved the technology of vaccine delivery via a cold-chain system in poorer countries, widely used for polio vaccines, and by expanding their policy to include disposable, self-destructive syringes. Steve Landry championed this innovation, after evidence showed that several thousand people died every year due to dirty syringes.[83]

The breakthrough success of IFFIm in reducing market volatility and providing a stable long-term financial platform for childhood inoculations belie the turbulent political machinations, and stakeholder tensions leading up to its launch. Within the corridors of power, all of the major stakeholders involved in GAVI were jockeying for position, all wanting the same thing – to be the recipient of the multibillion-dollar fund. Some of the rivalry originated from the Gates Foundation's own business practice of imposing a complex, lattice-like financial matrix, interlinking the GAVI network to safeguard the tax-exempt status of the $750 million in accordance with the 501(c) 3 code of the US internal revenue code. This involved establishing The Vaccine Fund under the presidency of Jacques-Francois Martin, with offices in Lyon, France and Washington, DC. This prestigious body acted as an intermediary to finance GAVI, oversee fundraising activities and build relationships with governments; in addition, Nelson Mandela, the world's most illustrious politician, chaired its Board. Some members of the Working Group and the secretariat felt hemmed in by The Vaccine Fund's micromanagement and wanted to unify the finance and the programme arms into one entity. Compounding the antipathies caused by this labyrinthine funding system, senior officials at the World Bank, WHO and UNICEF were feeling increasingly emasculated by GAVI and sought to impose their own agencies' control of how future monies are spent.[84] The inherent tensions and resentments within the alliance came to head at a meeting held at 66 Avenue d'léana, the Paris office of the World Bank. According to Godal the occasion was, 'the darkest day of my time at GAVI'.[85] The foreboding was understandable given that the representatives of the World Bank, UNICEF, WHO, all lined up and forcefully told Godal that they wanted to be the recipient of the IFFIm money. Carol Bellamy was particularly vociferous in her criticism of GAVI and by implication Godal as its de facto CEO – for having pushed UNICEF aside from its historic position, at the gravitational centre of immunisation.[86] Godal had a gift for being the unseen mover of events,[87] and the diplomatic skills to sidestep and smooth over political disagreements that would dangerously divide the partners. He was not known for his small talk, which proved useful when the stakes were so high and the temperature in the room was rising; his skills were in making strategic contacts at the highest echelons of politics and then making simple, convincing arguments.

> As usual in those situations, I kept my head down as I knew it would be up to Gordon Brown to make a decision. I also knew that he had been in discussions with the Gates Foundation and they were attracted by the lean and effective operations of GAVI, compared to the bloated bureaucracies of the other organisations. Soon after the meeting at the World Bank offices, Gordon Brown took the decision that GAVI would be the recipient of the IFFIm funds.[88]

Just four years after Bill Gates signed the cheque for $750 million, he announced that it was the best investment he had ever made.[89]

One year later, in 2004, Patty Stonesifer discovered that it was possible to send funds directly from the Foundation to the GAVI account at UNICEF without the need of an intermediary to protect its charitable status under the 501(c) 3 code regulations. This removed the need for The Vaccine Fund, which was absorbed into GAVI, while some of its Board members, including Jens Stoltenberg, joined the enlarged GAVI Board. Within five years, power had coalesced around Godal, the executive secretary of GAVI. As many of his colleagues would attest, there is a modesty to Godal,[90] but through the compelling mix of self-confidence, his low-key, yet steadfast, goal-orientated character and his unique ties to the Director-General of the WHO, Gro Harlem Brundtland, he converted the seemingly feeble position of executive secretary into being the leader of the alliance.[91] During his tenure, GAVI became one of the power hitters in global health; intrinsically, his skill was at starting things, sustaining the spark, building systems, and pushing through obstacles to get the programme to immunise the world's children off the ground and make it succeed. Moreover, the public–private model that GAVI pioneered has now become commonplace not only in health but also across the field of development, where the historical squeamishness of this sector to the profit-motive ethic of the private sector has dissipated in the era of the Millennium Development Goals. Of course, organisations need to mature; they need to build computer systems, develop rules and regulations, and governance and implement ways of doing things. In 2003, Godal was asked by the Gates Foundation to reapply for his position within GAVI – others applied for the post – at the interview he made it known that he would only stay in post for a further two years. Godal believed that the subsequent transition into maturity should be carried out by others, and in 2005, he stepped down from his role and was succeeded by the health systems specialist, Julian Lob-Levyt.

It would be, however, a mistake to think that the increased rates of childhood immunisation under GAVI formed a smooth and trouble-free curve of progress – there were some unforeseen consequences of policy decisions. In 2006, Chris Murray and his colleagues at the Institute of Health Metrics published a devastating paper in *The Lancet*[92] showing that there was a discrepancy between countries' official reports of WHO and UNICEF estimates compared to surveys using all available data. The study revealed that GAVI's immunisation services support payments of $20 paid per additional child immunised encouraged over-reporting, and that, 'immunisation coverage has improved more gradually and not to the level suggested'.[93] Godal was 'angry'[94] when he read the article because in the spirit of the public sector, he had helped to introduce a performance payment, and knew that the over-reporting of performance was a real possibility.

> Quite soon, we discovered that the records at the health centres could contain several pages with the exact same handwriting and thereby making us suspicious that the numbers were made up. We therefore started to plan for a modification, by which one would move the survey down to the village level.[95]

The article forcefully made the case for independent and contestable monitoring of health indicators in an era of global initiatives that are target-orientated and disburse funds based on performance. The relationship between Chris Murray and Tore Godal goes back a long way and while the article initially caused some friction; the statistical scrutiny acted as a force for good in the opinion of Chris Murray.

> The paper in *The Lancet* had a lot of influence on Tore and on GAVI. Initially it wasn't welcomed. But we found lower vaccine coverage in many countries than what was being officially recorded. We had a long-running discussion with Tore about this, but the incentive payment part was based on the idea that countries would be honest, but of course, when there is a financial incentive to gain numbers; one knows from many settings that people cheat the system. We should not be surprised if people exaggerate, whether intentionally or unintentionally. To Tore's credit, I think the programme corrected a lot in how they paid money to countries and got them to extend vaccine coverage. Of course, the great contribution of GAVI has been the financing of new vaccines. So, when rotavirus and pneumococcal conjugate vaccines got recommended the speed with which countries adopted those was dramatically faster because of GAVI.[96]

In 2013, many years after his direct association with GAVI, Paul Fife found himself once again working with the formidable Carol Bellamy. Bellamy was then the Chair of the Global Partnership for Education (GPE), and Fife was the head of a governance group within the GPE; one afternoon Carol Bellamy called him into her office.

> She said to me: '*We must be like GAVI!*' I started laughing and said something like, 'Carol when we worked with GAVI, UNICEF had to be dragged into the GAVI partnership'. Because GAVI was established because UNICEF and WHO had dropped the ball on immunisation after 1990. Carol, I think had an admiration for Tore but she was irritated that he was always ahead of us and so I thought it was hilarious when a few years later she said '*We must be like GAVI*'. What is clear is that it has always been better, and I am speaking about being on another team. It is always better to be on Tore's team than being on the opposition.[97]

In New York City, on Friday 20 September 2019 GAVI, the Vaccine Alliance (as it is now known) was presented with the Lasker-Bloomberg Public Service Awarded for providing sustained access to childhood vaccines around the globe, thus saving millions of lives and for highlighting the power of immunisation to prevent disease. The Lasker Prize is the US equivalent of the Nobel Prize. Gro Harlem Brundtland and Tore Godal attended the ceremony, together with

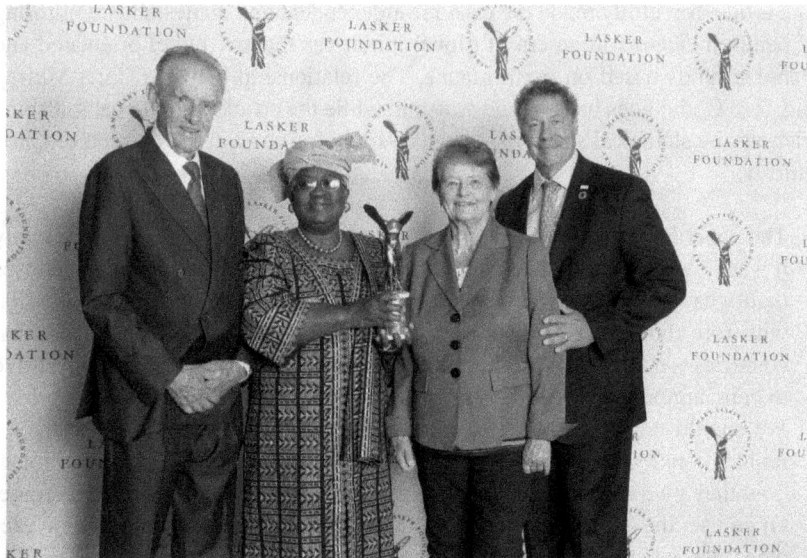

Figure 4.2 On Friday 20 September 2019, GAVI, the Vaccine Alliance was presented
with the Lasker-Bloomberg Public Service Award for providing access to
childhood vaccines. The prize was accepted at a ceremony in New York
City by (from left to right) Tore Godal, GAVI board member Ngozi Okonjo-
Iweala, Gro Harlem Brundtland and Seth Berkley.

Source: Courtesy of The Lasker Foundation.

GAVI board member Ngozi Okonjo-Iweala, now the Director-General of the
World Trade Organization, and Seth Berkeley, who became GAVI's CEO in
2011, accepted the prize. In his acceptance speech, Berkeley told the audience
that over the previous 19 years of its existence GAVI had helped to vaccinate
more than 760 million children and saved over 13 million lives in 73 countries.
He added that the ability to introduce new vaccines quickly against meningitis
and other infectious diseases equitably had been GAVI's greatest achievement.
In conclusion, he said that GAVI had become somewhat anonymous in its own
history, described by some as global health's best-kept secret: 'Well now I guess
thanks to you, that secret is finally out'.[98] Within two decades the leadership of
GAVI, the Vaccine Alliance had become a global reference point.

At the same ceremony, the Lasker-DeBakey Clinical Medical Research Award
honoured three distinguished scientists – H. Michael Shephard, Dennis J. Salmon
and Alex Ullrich – who collectively invented Herceptin, the first monoclonal
antibody that blocks a cancer-causing protein, and developed into a life-saving
therapy for women with breast cancer. During his acceptance speech, Michael
Shephard struck a philosophical chord when he said, 'we need more dreamers,

being a dreamer is a good thing in science'. He is right. It was the dreamers at the Bellagio meetings whose vision for childhood immunisation had been vindicated, the long odds had been overcome, and a global common good, to protect vulnerable children across the world, had been set in train.

Notes

1. Interview with Richard Horton, August 2020.
2. M. B. A. Oldstone, *Viruses, Plagues, & History: Past, Present, and Future* (Oxford: Oxford University Press, 2010), p. 53.
3. M. B. A. Oldstone, *Viruses, Plagues, & History: Past, Present, and Future* (Oxford: Oxford University Press, 2010), p. 56.
4. W. Muraskin, *Crusade to Immunize the World's Children* (Los Angeles: Global Bio-business Books: University of Southern California, 2005), p. xiii.
5. K. S. Warren, A. F. Mahmoud (eds.), *Tropical and Geographical Medicine* (New York: MC Graw-Hill Book Company, 1984).
6. G. Walt, P. Vaughan, *An Introduction to Primary Health Care Approach in Developing Countries: A Review With Selected Annotated References* (London: Ross Institute of Tropical Hygiene publ. no. 13, 1981).
7. J. Goodfield, *A Chance to Live: The Heroic Story of the Global Campaign to Immunise the World's Children* (New York: Macmillan, 1990), p. 3.
8. Kenneth Warren, Director of Health Sciences at the Rockefeller Foundation, viewed Alma-Ata as a distraction from finding the most efficient way of improving the life expectancy and reducing the suffering of the world's poorest people. In 1979, Warren and his colleague, Julia Walsh wrote a paper titled 'Selective primary health care: an interim strategy for disease control in developing countries' published in the *New England Journal of Medicine*. The article marked a departure from the traditional indicators, such as life expectancy at birth and infant mortality, to look at specific causes of death. In the paper, the major infectious diseases of the less developed world were placed in the order of their importance based on the number of deaths produced, and the disabilities caused, ranging from weakness and inability to work and learn to crippling and disfigurement. This exercise had never been carried out before, and it showed that the two most devastating health problems in the developing world were diarrheal diseases and respiratory infections of infants and young children, each of which was responsible for five million to ten million deaths per year. The authors advocated, 'instituting selective primary health care directed at preventing or treating those few diseases responsible for the greatest mortality in less developed areas and for which interventions of proven high efficacy exist'.
9. J. A. Walsh, K. S. Warren, "Selective primary health care: An interim strategy for disease control in the developing countries", *New England Journal of Medicine*, 1979, 301 (18), pp. 967–974.
10. W. H. Foege, *The Task Force for Child Survival: Secrets of Successful Coalitions* (Baltimore: Johns Hopkins University Press, 2018), p. 14.
11. Interview with Bill Foege, March 2020.
12. Interview with Bill Foege, March 2020.
13. Gro Harlem Brundtland, *Madam Prime Minister: A Life in Power and Politics* (New York: Farrar, Strauss and Giroux, 2002), p. 465.
14. *The New York Times*, "Indifference toward vaccinating the poor", Editorial, Monday, 21 January 2002, A14.
15. Interview with Seth Berkley, November 2019.

16. Gro Harlem Brundtland, Director General Elect, The World Health Organization. Speech to the 51st World Health Assembly, Geneva, 13 May 1998, p. 2.
17. C. Keating, *Kenneth Warren and the Great Neglected Diseases of Mankind Programme: The Transformation of Geographical Medicine in the US and Beyond* (New York: Springer, 2017).
18. Interview with Tim Evans, January 2020.
19. Herb Pigman was a former director of Rotary International Task Force for the Polio-Plus Program. The Task Force was launched by Rotary's child immunization operation throughout Asia, the Pacific, Latin America and Africa. By 1993, more than 500 million children in developing countries had been immunised against polio. At one time, Rotary International bought all of the polio vaccines in the world and had branches that raised money in over one hundred countries.
20. Interview with Barry Bloom, October 2020.
21. Interview with Tim Evans, January 2020.
22. Interview with Tim Evans, January 2020.
23. Interview with Tim Evans, January 2020.
24. W. Muraskin, *Crusade to Immunize the World's Children* (Los Angeles: Global Biobusiness Books: University of Southern California, 2005), p. 134.
25. Interview with Dean Jamison, April 2020.
26. The group included Jonas Gahr Store of WHO, Dave de Ferranti and Chris Lovelace of the World Bank, Jacque-Francois Martin, Mark Kane representing the Gates Foundation, and David Alnwick of UNICEF.
27. The membership included Amie Batson of the World Bank, Suomi Sakai of UNICEF, Mike Levine of the Rockefeller Foundation, Michel Zaffran of WHO and Jacques-Francois Martin.
28. W. Muraskin, *Crusade to Immunize the World's Children* (Los Angeles: Global Biobusiness Books: University of Southern California, 2005), p. 136.
29. Interview with Tore Godal, August 2018.
30. Interview with Tore Godal, August 2018.
31. Interview with Seth Berkley, November 2019.
32. Interview with Helga Fogstead, August 2020.
33. Interview with Tim Evans, January 2020.
34. Interview with Carol Bellamy, April 2020.
35. J. N. Smith, *Epic Measures: One Doctor: Seven Billion Patients* (New York: Harper Collins, 2015), p. 144.
36. J. N. Smith, *Epic Measures: One Doctor: Seven Billion Patients* (New York: Harper Collins, 2015), p. 144.
37. J. H. L. Playfair, in I. M. Roitt (ed.), *Immune Intervention: New Trends in Vaccines*, vol. 1 (London: Academic Press, 1984), p. 1.
38. Interview with Seth Berkley, November 2019.
39. Obituary of James Wolfensohn, by Jurek Martin and Martin Wolf, *The Financial Times Weekend*, 28–29 November 2020, p. 8.
40. Interview with Tim Evans, January 2020.
41. Gustav Nossal was chair of the influential Scientific Advisory Group of Experts (SAGE), which oversaw both the WHO's Global Programme on Vaccines and the Children's Vaccine Initiative.
42. Gordon Perkin, Gordon Duncan and Richard Mahoney founded PATH (Program for Appropriate Technology in Health) in 1977, with a focus on family planning. It later expanded into vaccines and immunisation, mother and child health, and emerging and epidemic diseases.
43. Interview with Barry Bloom, October 2020.

44. Interview with Tore Godal, August 2018.
45. Interview with Tore Godal, August 2018.
46. Interview with Bo Stenson, October 2020.
47. Interview with Seth Berkley, November 2019.
48. A. Crump, "Tore Godal: Pragmatic optimist championing global public health", *Trends in Parasitology*, 2006, 22 (8), p. 381.
49. Interview with Sir Gustav Nossal, October 2019.
50. Interview with Amie Batson, August 2020.
51. Interview with Amie Batson, August 2020.
52. Email communication from Jeff Sachs, October 2020.
53. Interview with Amie Batson, August 2020.
54. Interview with Tore Godal, November 2019.
55. Interview with Bo Stenson, November 2020.
56. Interview with Bo Stenson, November 2020.
57. Interview with Lisa Jacobs, November 2020.
58. Interview with Lisa Jacobs, November 2020.
59. Interview with Bo Stenson, November 2020.
60. Interview with Tore Godal, August 2018.
61. Interview with Jens Stoltenberg, July 2019.
62. Stoltenberg wished it could have been more, but it was a time of austerity, and if one sector got an increase, it necessitated financial cuts elsewhere.
63. Throughout this period, Jonas Gahr Støre was working behind the scenes, and it was him that suggested to Godal that Jens Stoltenberg should be given a seat on the GAVI board.
64. S. Boseley, "Norway's Prime Minister Jens Stoltenberg: Leader on MDG 4", *The Lancet*, 22 September 2007, 370, p. 1027.
65. S. Boseley, "Norway's Prime Minister Jens Stoltenberg: Leader on MDG 4", *The Lancet*, 22 September 2007, 370, p. 1027.
66. Interview with Jens Stoltenberg, July 2020.
67. During 2003–2006, approximately 15.4 million children in China-GAVI project received the three-dose HepB series, preventing an estimated 1.47 million chronic HBV infections in children and 265,000 future deaths attributable to chronic HBV infection.
68. Interview with Tore Godal, August 2018.
69. Interview with Tore Godal, August 2018.
70. Interview with Viroj Tangcharoensathien, November 2020.
71. Interview with Alice Albright, November 2020.
72. Interview with Violaine Mitchell, June 2020.
73. Interview with Paul Fife, February 2020.
74. Interview with Steve Landry, June 2020.
75. Interview with Violaine Mitchell, June 2020.
76. Interview with Amie Batson, August 2020.
77. Interview with Tore Godal, December 2020.
78. Personnel communication, Gordon Brown. Email April 2020.
79. Interview with Alice Albright, November 2020.
80. In 2019, Michael Kremer was jointly awarded the Nobel Memorial Prize in Economics, together with Esther Duflo and Abhijit Banerjee 'for their experimental approach to alleviating poverty'.
81. Interview with Alice Albright, November 2020.
82. Interview with Seth Berkley, November 2019.
83. Interview with Tore Godal, August 2018.

84. Interview with Steve Landry, June 2020.
85. Interview with Tore Godal, August 2018.
86. Interview with Violaine Mitchell, June 2020.
87. W. Muraskin, *Crusade to Immunize the World's Children* (Los Angeles: Global Bio-business Books: University of Southern California, 2005), p. 215.
88. Interview with Tore Godal, August 2018.
89. Interview with Seth Berkley, November 2019.
90. Interview with Chris Murray, February 2019.
91. W. Muraskin, *Crusade to Immunize the World's Children* (Los Angeles: Global Bio-business Books: University of Southern California, 2005), p. 215.
92. S. S. Lim, D. B. Stein, A. Charrow, C. J. L. Murray, "Tracking progress towards universal childhood immunisation and the impact of global initiatives: A systematic analysis of three-dose diphtheria, tetanus, and pertussis immunisation coverage", *Lancet*, 2008, 372, pp. 2031–2046.
93. S. S. Lim, D. B. Stein, A. Charrow, C. J. L. Murray, "Tracking progress towards universal childhood immunisation and the impact of global initiatives: A systematic analysis of three-dose diphtheria, tetanus, and pertussis immunisation coverage", *Lancet*, 2008, 372, p. 2031.
94. Interview with Tore Godal, August 2018.
95. Interview with Tore Godal, August 2018.
96. Interview with Chris Murray, February 2019.
97. Interview with Paul Fife, February 2020.
98. Interview with Seth Berkley, November 2019.

5 Maternal and Child Health

The Great Leap Forward

Tore Godal is the most expensive Norwegian in history.

Jens Stoltenberg[1]

Millennium Development Goals 2015

Just as in politics, science and art, personalities shape global health. Yet the ability of even the most influential people to effect levels of mortality in low-income countries is contingent upon the difficult art, science and politics of setting cost-effective health priorities in a systematic manner.[2] At the beginning of the twenty-first century, a profound conversion marked a new momentum for global health innovation. In September 2000, world leaders gathered at the United Nations in New York to reaffirm their commitment to a more peaceful, prosperous and just world. The Millennium Declaration Development Goals were an audacious set of 8 goals and 21 incremental targets to reduce extreme poverty and hunger; empower women; and combat HIV/AIDS, malaria and other diseases.[3] The MDGs encouraged, among other things, peace and disarmament, development and poverty eradication, and addressing the 'special needs of Africa' all of which were certainly honourable objectives, but how were those organisations and individuals that are on the frontline against extreme poverty, injustice and ill-health to be helped in a meaningful way? This was one of the questions that the Prime Minister of Norway, Jens Stoltenberg, asked himself as he flew home to Oslo from New York in September 2000. He knew that while he had participated in a meeting that had the potential to be a decisive moment in global health, at the same time, he was troubled that a great opportunity might be lost. 'Eradicating deadly diseases such as malaria and HIV/AIDS and reducing childhood mortality and levels of poverty were very good goals', mused the concerned politician, 'but I also thought that the Millennium Development Goals would probably end up like another one of those international meetings where everyone has forgotten what they agreed upon when they are back at home'.[4] At the time, Stoltenberg was the political leader of a country with a population of just 4.5 million, but due

DOI: 10.4324/9781003363859-6

to its wealth and commitment to multilateralism, Norway was the seventh largest donor to the UN, which allowed it to have a big impact on the content and design of global health planning. This powerful leadership role, signposting the way forward for other donor nations to follow, saw Norway become the first country to pledge financial support for the Global Alliance for Vaccines and Immunisation (GAVI) Alliance, and encouraged in Stoltenberg a long-term ambition to make the drive for improved global health a central platform of his country's foreign policy.[5]

In addition to his political powerbase,[6] Stoltenberg had had a stellar academic career – he was awarded the best ever degree in economics from the University of Oslo, and went onto become one of the country's leading statisticians, refining his skills as a researcher at the Central Bureau of Statistics in the 1980s. This experience gave him a numerical understanding of the global burden of disease metrics (DALYs), demography and a proficiency in cost-effective analysis – collectively the indispensable tools required for setting health priorities in a systematic way. Importantly, Stoltenberg held deep-seated moral views regarding the responsibilities of wealthy countries to less wealthy ones, and his forte as a politician was combining a clear moral purpose with a mastery of technical minutiae. It was not, however, a monocausal chain of events that led to his call to action; rather, it was a combination of forces and the influence of three key individuals: first, Gro Harlem Brundtland, who brought Stoltenberg into her government in 1990 as State Secretary at the Ministry of Environment, second, his chief of staff, the intellectual powerhouse, Jonas Gahr Støre, and finally, Tore Godal. From Brundtland, the country's first woman prime minister and widely known as 'the mother of the nation', the people of Norway – and Stoltenberg – had been given a physician's perspective on health and political issues, and in her extremely rational approach to politics she delivered diagnoses and prescribed remedies to social ills. Jonas Ghar Støre had been Brundtland's special advisor, and as Chief of Staff at WHO in Geneva from 1998 to 2000, the brilliant conceptual thinker was constantly searching for new ways in which a small country like Norway could make a big difference on the world stage. He was not alone in this mission. To some global health specialists,[7] the crucial moment for UN Millennium Goals 4 and 5 occurred in March 2000, when Tore Godal and Jens Stoltenberg met for the first time. In the spring of 2000, Godal was a powerful figure in global health; he was Executive Secretary of (GAVI) and had made strategic contacts at the highest echelons of world politics, establishing a reputation for making simple and convincing arguments for reducing preventable childhood deaths. His talent, according to one UN expert, was being able to 'read people extremely well',[8] and then convey the ethical and economic importance of an idea with such compassion and feeling that his conviction inspired an awakening in others to join his cause. On this occasion, his big picture vision, delivered in a direct and concise style, appealed greatly to the quantitative-minded, data-driven, Stoltenberg.

Tore was a medical doctor and I was an economist and while I knew something about the dangers of malaria, I didn't have a clue about the death toll from measles. He explained how vaccines worked. I learned a lot about rotavirus, and why we had not been able to eradicate polio. . . . We would sit together for hours on a plane and he regarded me as a type of student of medicine. I would ask questions and I loved listening to him talk about research, and about how vaccines were a cheap and effective tool against many diseases.[9]

Under Godal's expert tutelage, Stoltenberg became a convert to the idea of vaccinating the most marginalised children around the globe. This was a transformational time in the history of science-based medicine, and the advent of the Bill and Melinda Gates Foundation revolutionised the funding of global public health issues, especially in the area of vaccines. The burgeoning dyad between public and private innovations was further galvanised in the form of a strong bond of friendship that developed between Stoltenberg and Bill Gates and their shared determination to do something in global health that mattered, and crucially, that was measurable. One of Godal's maxims is, 'if you want real progress then you have to find real problems',[10] and childhood mortality was one of the most intractable global health problems of the new millennium. Godal viewed science as a potential force for social change by its ability to intervene and control nature in the interests of humanity. His thinking and scientific attitude had been influenced by one of his immunological heroes, Peter Medawar, who had sent a warm letter welcoming Godal to the National Institute for Medical Research, in the late 1960s. Medawar saw medical research as being 'the art of the soluble',[11] meaning that there seems to be a certain time when some biomedical questions are especially ripe for answering, whereas other problems remain stubbornly elusive, intractable and out of reach. Medawar believed that good scientists study the most important problems that they think they can solve. Fortunately, Godal knew that he had found a political ally in Stoltenberg who, for ethical and developmental reasons, wanted good health to be more evenly distributed, and not something that was largely confined to populations living in the rich developed world.

Achieving the health Millennium Development Goals – reducing child mortality; improving maternal health; and combating HIV/AIDS, malaria and other diseases – by 2015 was always going to be difficult,[12] but in 2001 the newly formed Godal-Stoltenberg alliance suffered a serious setback. In the parliamentary elections of 10 September 2001, the Norwegian electorate delivered the Labour Party one of its worst ever results, winning less than a quarter of all the votes cast. Stoltenberg's brief tenure as prime minister was over, but during his subsequent four years in opposition he cultivated a devotion to global health, by becoming a member of the board of The Vaccine Fund with Nelson Mandela as Chair and serving as a director of GAVI. During this time, he also gained some first-hand experience of a vaccine rollout in countries with resource poor health systems.

> I travelled with GAVI to Pakistan and Senegal. It was a magical experience to give my first polio vaccine by dropping a few drops on the tongue of an African child in rural Senegal. At the simple health station there was a long queue of girls in their late teens, they each brought their little child. One by one they came into the small office, where there was a light bulb in the ceiling, a modest writing desk and a couple of chairs.[13]

This experience convinced Stoltenberg, who at the time was a father of small children, that it was a moral obligation to help others, and that saving the life of the child was both cost-effective and beneficial to the entire nation. As an economist, he knew that healthy children participate in the development of a country as parents spend less time nursing sick and dying children and more on creating income from productive work. This served to reinforce in Stoltenberg's mind what he had learned from Godal; that by eliminating poverty causing diseases in a cost-effective way, societies could be changed.

The MDG Push on Maternal and Child Health

When a rejuvenated Labour Party won the general election in September 2005, Jens Stoltenberg once again became prime minister, leading a coalition government made up of other progressive parties.[14] Stoltenberg's closest advisers were the Foreign Minister, Jonas Gahr Støre and State Secretary, Morten Wetland. Their task was to identify a platform for the new Prime Minister that would elevate Norway as a power broker and catalyst in the international arena for global health investment. In the days of September and October 2005, one question concentrated their minds – how does a small country like Norway punch above its weight in the global health arena? Complex discussions centred on what they had learnt from Godal, Brundtland and others in the preceding years about setting health priorities that mattered and were measurable. The concepts of 'making a difference' and 'the measurement of health systems performance' were much in the spirit of the time since the publication of The World Health Report 2000 *Health Systems: Improving Performance*. In her introduction to the report, the Director-General, Gro Harlem Brundtland wrote, 'I hope this report will help policymakers to make wise choices. If they do so, substantial gains will be possible for all countries, and the poor will be the principal beneficiaries'. Gahr Støre, Wetland and Stoltenberg knew that Brundtland relied heavily on the advice of Tore Godal when it came to global health thinking, and the WHO Report *Health Systems: Improving Performance* put the focus 'on results' and 'measurement of outcomes'. The editor-in-chief of *The Lancet*, Richard Horton, believes the report is a profoundly important document in the history of the WHO.

It provided conceptual insights into the complex factors that explain how health systems perform, and offered practical advice on how to assess performance and achieve improvements with available resources. Suddenly WHO had got into the business of measuring the effectiveness of health systems and that had never happened before.[15]

Measurement and cost-effectiveness were going to be essential components for the new administrations global health strategy. For his part, Stoltenberg was critical of how wasteful some parts of the Norwegian aid programme had been selected. For too long, donor countries like Norway gave away large amounts of un-earmarked funds, and therefore there was no measurable return on spending. Operationally, this was unacceptable to Stoltenberg's arithmetically leaning world view. In its place, he wanted an international aid programme that was orientated towards results in the field. One of the most celebrated advocates of results-based financing in global public health policy was the indefatigable Godal, who embedded this ideal into GAVI's operational philosophy and later into the health metrics that underpinned the funding principles of the World Bank.[16] In this way, Godal's influence on performance-based financing for health in developing countries proved to be both subtle and indelible.

Within Stoltenberg's inner-circle of political advisors, the guidance was unambiguous: 'My recommendation to Jens', recalled Jonas Ghar Støre,

was that this is your opportunity. As the Prime Minister of Norway, you can take the lead in global health, but you will need quality advice. Therefore, we recruited Tore as special advisor to the PM, in the PM's office, which had never happened before. No PM had ever had an advisor on global public health.[17]

Godal's analytical strength and innovative mind-set gave him the ability to think strategically and ensure the use of evidence when implementing political decisions. This combination linking research, policy and operations was, in the opinion of Bard Vegar Solhjell, Director-General of Norad (The Norwegian Agency for Development Cooperation), 'the reason Jonas Ghar Støre brought Tore in to advise Jens. It was for his operational brain'.[18] However, before Godal could take up his post on the fifteenth floor of the tower block housing the prime minister's office – which featured vast steel doors that could snap closed in the event of a terrorist attack – two outstanding issues needed to be resolved. First, Godal may have known his way around the labyrinthine workings of the international technocracies of the UN and WHO, but before confirming his appointment, the State Secretary, Morten Wetland first had to navigate a safe passage through the intransigence of the Norwegian bureaucracy.

Some of the puritans in the bureaucracy said, 'you have to have a competition for such a post', which I thought was completely ridiculous. You could only find one person on the planet that had the qualifications, and that was Tore. [Nonetheless], we did have a competition and I more or less copy and pasted Tore's CV into the advertisement, which said 'anyone who corresponds to these requirements is welcome to apply.[19]

One other person did apply. Second, and closer to home, before Godal could to take up this powerful role in Norwegian politics, he had to persuade his Australian born wife, Ann, to uproot her life, leave their bucolic home near Geneva and relocate to Oslo. Godal's first marriage to Kari had ended in divorce, and both Ann and Tore arrived independently in Geneva in 1986 to work at the World Health Organization. In the early 1990s, they met, fell in love and married in 1993. Tore had found, in the words of his colleague Helga Fogstad, 'the jewel and diamond in his life'.[20] In 1998, when Brundtland won the election to become Director-General of the WHO, Ann Kern-Godal became the head of her administration. Another historical coincidence, and one that may have made Ann more amenable to moving to Oslo, was that earlier in her career as a health administrator, she had worked in the office of the Australian Prime Minister. Within weeks, they moved their collective centre of gravity to Oslo, and Godal became Stoltenberg's special adviser in November 2005.

Godal's strategic thinking became immediately apparent on the political priorities of the new administration. The first speech Stoltenberg gave as Prime Minister in 2005 was titled 'Vaccination against poverty', and later that year, in recognition of his work as Board member of the Global Alliance for Vaccines and Immunisation, Stoltenberg received the Children's Health Award. The GAVI model delivered the proof-of-concept evidence that childhood vaccination saved lives, and that 'health' could translate directly into 'wealth', persuaded Stoltenberg that spending billions of dollars on a global health programme to reduce child mortality was going to make a difference. 'I was convinced', Stoltenberg, reminisced 15 years later,

> by the value of vaccines both as an economist because it was extremely cost-effective, and as a politician, because I could communicate to the tax-payers of Norway that their money is being spent in an extremely cost-effective way, achieving a huge effect for a low cost.[21]

In 2005, as Godal provided the strategic direction that put Norway in the forefront of the global campaign for childhood vaccination (MDG 4), UN Secretary-General, Kofi Annan complained that governments around the world were not taking the MDGs seriously. Working just below the surface of Norwegian politics, and having greater levels of autonomy than many government ministers,[22] Godal according to Stoltenberg 'was always looking for opportunities for how we can be of influence, and how we can change the world'.[23] Godal held no formal political position within the government; his role was that of an adviser on global public health, but for more than a decade, his habitat was the environs of political power. Nonetheless, while Godal was an integral part of a network of influential groups across the globe, the problem he faced, according to Suprotik Basu, who at the time was a public health specialist at the World Bank, was that, 'health was barely at the table in the early 2000s'.[24] Godal's concern was for the vulnerability of people who do not have health care and his ambitious goal was to protect the most marginalised children, resuscitate interest in MDG 4 and develop new health priorities that were going to be good for the poorest of the poor. This would only be successful if he could deploy his newfound political influence, and by bringing others along with him. The objective was to develop a policy that over time would start to lead a sustainable life of its own. Of course, politics is a bruising environment in which to operate, and luckily for Godal, he had more allies than adversaries within Norwegian political circles. In the forefront of his defence from reactionary elements was State Secretary, Morten Wetland. As an experienced, and politically astute diplomat, he pre-emptively manoeuvred to counteract any attempts to obfuscate or delay the governments, and de facto, Godal's global health policies. 'My role was to establish an anti-aircraft gun on top of the prime minister's office and shoot down any incoming missiles that would prevent Tore from doing an effective job and to protect him against the bureaucratic forces'.[25] Godal is renowned for his tenacity and mild demeanour, and while he recognised the indispensability of political power, he would collaborate with *any* politician or *any* officeholder in order to implement his vision to advance the health of the global poor. In this sense, he saw leadership not as a power role but as one of service and enabling others. He cared deeply about evidence-based policies and about results at the country level, and was little interested in the vanity around it. Of course, he wanted others to embrace *his* idea, and in return, he offered them the limelight and kudos of the big stage, perhaps at the UN General Assembly in New York City, or the WHO in Geneva, where they could campaign and receive the admiration for what may have become *their* innovative idea. Another physician operating on the fulcrum of the politics-health axis is Richard Horton, who has an understandable admiration for his friend's capacity to pole-vault ideas up the global health agenda.

> Tore is a big ideas guy; he sees the bigger picture and the political opportunity. He likes being close to power; and he is made of steel in terms of his grit and determination to get something done. And, he has a way of speaking that is very direct, but that is the Norwegian way, to be very direct. The other thing is that he is an extraordinary nice man.[26]

This outward civility was genuine and wholehearted, but once Godal had settled on a course of action, he was utterly tenacious in assembling a coalition to ensure its success. He had, what Suprotik Basu, describes as 'sharp elbows' and uses 'politics aggressively';[27] moreover, when someone in the Norwegian government, civil service or the media picked up the telephone and heard Tore Godal's voice, no one was under any illusions, when he spoke, they were listening to the views of the prime minister.

The Norway India Partnership Initiative (NIPI)

Ideas in global health can have a distinct lineage that reflect and correspond to the same evolutionary chronology as the study of peoples, cultures and societies. Thus, understanding the concept of evidence-based medicine and the influence of social Darwinism animate the historical development and operational drive to improve maternal health care (MDG 5). Having been fortified in his thinking by the establishment of The Partnership for Maternal, New Born and Child Health (PMNCH) in 2005 – and hosted at the WHO in Geneva – Godal sought to expand the reach of the Stoltenberg government's commitment with a global campaign to improve maternal health. This seemed a logical step as the 'appalling mortality figures for children and pregnant women',[28] would continue unless countries, aid agencies and development partners intensified their efforts. Besides, in Godal's mind, there was an ontological relationship between MDGs 4 and 5 – one could not exist, in developmental terms, without the other. Child health was inseparable from maternal health, but as a leading proponent of the results-based finance school of thought, he knew that 'the data and measurement of maternal health posed a challenge'.[29] In this context, seeking to reproduce the cost-effectiveness metric of vaccines-to-lives-saved was an operational impediment. Clearly, the definition of evidence-based policies would need to be etymologically stretched to encompass a longer time period, to include the strengthening of countries' health systems as a whole and making and delivering long-term commitments.[30]

Philosophically, maternal health was a challenge to the prevailing world view of *results-based finance*, and as Godal was a leading proponent of the system, he increasingly became the embodiment of that tension. At the time, Helga Fogstad was responsible for Norad's (Norwegian Agency for Development Cooperation) portfolio for global health, to promote the rapid scale-up of proven cost-effective interventions and witnessed at first hand Godal's methodological dilemma.

> Tore wasn't totally convinced about maternal and child health. He understood the value of vaccination, but he needed to be convinced that maternal health would benefit the child and the dyad between mother and newborn. . . . Then to go for a systems approach, strengthening the systems in a very practical way.[31]

Operationally, the objective for Godal was to get the greatest value for money spent, and while he believed absolutely in the policy of maternal health, the reality was that MDG5 was not going to be quantifiable in the same metric timeframe as childhood vaccination (MDG4). Early in 2006, at a global health meeting at the Norwegian embassy in London, Godal had a conversation with Chris Murray and asked if it possible to accurately measure 'progress' in MDG 5 and Murray's reply was a reassuring 'yes'. Also, closer to home, Jen's Stoltenberg's mother, Karin, while working for the Norwegian Agency for Development Cooperation had supported the ideals of equity and women's health. Family history, the economics of health metrics and evaluation, and political culture were beginning to coalesce. Building a commitment and putting more resources into the policy clearly struck a resonant chord with the Norwegian people as witnessed by Godal. 'People spontaneously clap when [Jens Stoltenberg] speaks about getting children in the third world vaccinated. People see it not as politics but as a kind of cause. It is something close to his heart'.[32] Politicians in Norway are answerable to their electorate, and clearly, there was a danger that their vaccine-orientated global health message, with its clear and explainable profile, might become diluted. However, Stoltenberg's government took that risk. Bringing a new life into the world can be a very dangerous event for many women, especially for those in developing countries, and while it clearly was a health issue, for Norway maternal health progressively became a question of equity, dignity and human rights.

In 2006, Norway needed to find partners to help create a momentum for maternal and child health. To that end, Godal and Morten Wetland went on a charm offensive to the German Chancellery and lobbied the Minister of Development Aid, explaining their new thinking about how to help the most disadvantaged. Wetland remembered the German federal government as being, 'a bit like a super-tanker, slow in turning. It took a while but it went well'.[33] Meanwhile, Godal was developing strategies, capitalising in Jens Stoltenberg's commitment to MDGs 4 and 5, and looked around relentlessly for what was missing 'in the existing global architecture of health aid'[34] to speed the train of maternal health. He found the answer in India. For many decades, Godal had studied primary health care provision in India, a country that was responsible for one-fifth of global health births and a quarter of neonatal deaths. During those years, through skilful groundwork, Godal established contacts at the very highest level in India, with politicians, technicians and public health figures that came to fruition in 2005 when he and Stoltenberg visited India to attend a GAVI Board meeting.

They were there as guests of the Permanent Secretary of Health, Prassanna Hota and Prime Minister Manmohan Singh, the first Sikh prime minister of India, and like Stoltenberg, an economist by training. Hota and Godal brought Singh and Stoltenberg together as part of a collaborative health programme called the Norwegian Indian Partnership Initiative (NIPI). One of the strategies the Norwegian delegation learnt from their Indian colleagues was that, as part of a pilot project in very poor regions, the government paid the medical costs of women who gave birth in clinics and hospitals. On a visit to a village in the state of Madhya Pradesh, in central India, they met a group of women that had benefited from the scheme. Jens Stoltenberg asked the women what the value of the scheme was to their lives and the reply was salutary. 'Yes, we benefited greatly, because for the first time we had a negotiating card to play with our mothers-in-law'.[35] The women went on to tell Godal and Stoltenberg that in the past, when their husbands went to their mothers asking if it was worthwhile for them to spend money on medical care for their wife in childbirth, the answer had invariably been along the lines of, 'No need my son. You were born at home and you're a wonderful boy'. The visit to Madhya Pradesh was instructive, as Godal saw it as a fine example of *results-based financing*, because the women received payment when they arrived at the clinic. 'I became excited', Godal recalled, 'when I saw how effective it was to offer financial incentives for women in poor rural communities in India to give birth to their babies safely in urban maternity clinics'.[36] This was the methodological and ethical breakthrough that Godal felt had been missing. In the years that followed, NIPI, funded by the Norwegian Ministry of Foreign Affairs, expanded its scalable interventions into the states of Bihar, Odisha, Madhya Pradesh and Rajasthan. When Prime Minister Modi succeeded Manmohan Singh, he was appalled that the maternal and child health of the neighbouring countries of Bangladesh and Nepal was better than that in India, and therefore made MDGs 4 and 5 a priority of his government. NIPI had a central role in shaping the policy that was adopted. NIPI's aim was, and continues to be, to provide strategic and innovative support to India's National Health Mission and reduce maternal, newborn and child mortality in the country. Now in its second decade of existence, NIPI[37] justifies its status as one the most impressive programmes in development cooperation.[38]

Historically, the early years of Jen Stoltenberg's second administration, with Godal constantly on his shoulder advising and encouraging him the whole time, constitutes a decisive period for the health Millennium Development Goals. Before Godal's arrival, Norad was in the opinion of its current Director-General, Bård Vegar Solhjell,

> rather a conservative institution development wise, and Tore was key to bringing results-based-financing into Norad. But, he was also important because he worked so well at the country level and with country programmes like NIPI. I sometimes wonder if that is forgotten, because of all the multilateral efforts that he was involved in. The Indian partnership was very important, and he is still well known in health circles in India, and it is one of many concrete programmes that had a good fit with the aid community and an institution like Norad.[39]

By showing that economic incentives encourage women to go to health facilities during their pregnancy and at childbirth, measures were implemented that save lives. Rather than a top-down directive, this was bottom-up enterprise, which enabled a country to decide its own health priority.

Women and Children First

With Godal acting as an intellectual echo chamber for maternal and child health, a concerted strategy emanated from the Norwegian government that created vibrations around the theme of the health Millennium Goals among the global health assemblage. The rapidly unfolding campaign signalled a commitment to finding better ways of achieving value for money and ensuring that the most vulnerable groups have access to essential services. In response to the World Health Report 2005: Make Every Mother and Child Count[40] and the accompanying policy briefs, Ministers of Health at the World Health Assembly passed a resolution putting maternal and child health at the top of their list of health priorities. Good intentions are no substitute for practical policies, and in 2006 when Godal rationally examined the MDG target of reducing the under-5 mortality rate by two-thirds by 2015, he quickly concluded that the existing global health system was incapable of reducing the millions of maternal and child deaths from preventable and treatable causes.[41] Clearly, a new global campaign was needed that would bring new money to the health MDGs and sustain interest in global health by demonstrating improved health outcomes. Capitalising on Stoltenberg's commitment and convening power, the Norwegian stratagem was to concentrate its attentions on the UN General Assembly in New York, where for a few days in late September, the multitude of heads of state, prime ministers and presidents, made the city the epicentre of global political power.

In a synchronized movement, Godal, Morten Wetland and Jonas Ghar Støre elevated MDGs 4 and 5 onto the world stage in 2006 by hosting a 'side event' for political leaders in the basement of UNICEF's headquarters. It was the genesis of a new network composed of the global political elite, led by Stoltenberg, which would grow into rambunctious 'spill-over' meetings at the UN General Assembly involving dozens of heads of state, including the presidents of Indonesia, Chile, Brazil and the prime ministers of the Netherlands, Pakistan and the United Kingdom. The close personal relationship between Gordon Brown, who became the UK prime minister in 2007, and Jens Stoltenberg proved decisive for the health-related MDGs. Brown was a passionate advocate for global action to fight poverty and create a more just world.[42] Health and development were the goals that both politicians shared, together with an enthusiasm for new financial mechanisms designed to channel more aid to developing countries. 'We established a good relationship with Gordon Brown', Morten Wetland recounted,

> Jens knew Gordon from the time they were both finance ministers, so we went in and out of No10 Downing Street and we shared responsibilities. 'If the UK did that part, then Norway will do this part'. We divided the work between ourselves and Tore could call the Secretary of State for International Development at any time.[43]

For his part, Godal respected Brown and Stoltenberg and believed that their shared background of Christian and socialist philanthropy galvanised a collective determination to lead a global drive to improve maternal and child health. 'They get on very well', Godal observed from his position within the upper levels of government, 'they collaborate closely. They are both doers. If they engage, something gets done'.[44]

How true that was. On 5 September 2007, Gordon Brown launched the International Health Partnerships – a global 'compact' for achieving the Health Millennium Goals – at a prestigious gathering at number 10 Downing Street.[45] This was a conscious act to close the gap between rhetoric and reality by improving the coordination of support for national health plans and bring together developing countries, international health organisations and major donor countries. Three weeks later, on 26 September, Jens Stoltenberg announced the Global Campaign for the Health Millennium Development Goals in New York City. The day after the presentation, some of the largest development assistance donors committed $9.7 billion in new finance for MDG 6 – combating HIV/AIDS, malaria and other diseases – in the period 2008–2010.[46] The campaign was Godal's brainchild and encompassed several actions that aimed to speed up progress on shared common principles.

- Countries decide their own health priorities and create national health plans to achieve them.
- More attention will be given to results, so that the money spent is linked to the results achieved in work on women and children's health.
- Aid agencies will work in ways that strengthen countries' health systems as a whole.
- Development partners to work together to coordinate their work in a newly established Heads of Health Agencies (the 'Health 8': World Health Organisation; World Bank; UNICEF; UN Fund for Population Activities; UNAIDS; GAVI Alliance; Global Fund to Fight AIDS, Tuberculosis and Malaria; and Bill & Melinda Gates Foundation).

Operating at the intersection of politics, science and global health, Godal created a network of political leaders, which included, among others, Barak Obama and Angela Merkel who campaigned for maternal and child health programmes. Additionally, he helped to create a Sherpa group of specialists that met twice a year, to generate ideas and proposals for the politicians. The idea was classic 'nudge theory', of positive reinforcement behaviour in operation. This meant that when a top politician agreed to make a one-page contribution to the publication on the health MDGs, a request would go down the hierarchical line of power, and ideas would percolate up through the layers of government designed to make the president or prime minister come across well on the world stage. Godal knew that this 'nudging' affected not only the leaders but also civil servants and ambitious politicians, to give more attention to MDGs 4 and 5.

Meanwhile, Norway's pledge to spend more money year-on-year on overseas aid began to recalibrate the funding dynamics of world health. During the intense budget negotiations between the three coalition parties of the Norwegian government, Godal received, a written message from Prime Minister Stoltenberg asking, 'If I could use an additional NOK 600 million per year?' After a moment's reflection, Godal selected his favoured means of communication, a Post-it Note, and sent this message back to his prime minister.[47] 'I could use 400 million next year and 600 million the years after that'. Godal had earmarked the money for a yet to be defined results-based financing scheme aimed at maternal and child health. It was a fortuitous decision, because in the autumn of 2007, he took a phone call from Amie Batson, a senior researcher at the World Bank in Washington, DC, and a friend from the early days of GAVI. Amie Batson needed help because she had hit a budgetary brick wall in her efforts to establish a new results-based financing project at the World Bank designed to speed progress towards the health commitments the world community had set for itself. At the beginning of the twenty-first century, the accepted dogma at the World Bank was that developing countries would borrow money to invest in infrastructure projects, education and hard assets, but not for health. However, Batson had been researching some innovative results-based financing projects in Argentina and thought there was a possibility of adapting the model to her health portfolio at the World Bank. Within a few years, Batson had succeeded in persuading the Gates Foundation to put up $100 million, and the money would be in a trust fund linked to World Bank loans, thereby reducing the borrowing costs for developing countries. Then after much careful planning and negotiation, disaster struck – the Gates Foundation told Batson that they were not going to fund the project.

> That is when I called Tore. When I told him that the Gates Foundation said they wouldn't fund it, he said, 'Okay, tell them we will fund half if they pay the other half'. This is vintage Tore. But, when I went back to the Gates Foundation with the offer they still said no. So, back I go to Tore . . . And he said, 'We're going to do it. This is too important. I'll come up with the $100 million'.

This was the backstory to how Norway became a first-mover, the first domino to put serious cash on the table, and the reward was harnessing a relationship and having influence within the highest strata of power at the World Bank. This funding stream for health later translated into the Health Results Innovation Trust Fund (HRITF), a very successful mechanism at the country level aimed at better outcomes for women and children. Funded by Norway and the United Kingdom, by 2014 it had $550 million at its disposal, supporting 36 programmes in 31 countries and saving millions of lives.[48]

Godal's pragmatism coupled with his discouragement of the cult of personality and *Jantaloven* world view gained him respect and trust from his colleagues. Because he did not promote his ideas in an egotistical way, but in the form of a global public good, his actions accorded admiration across the political spectrum in Norway. The relentless pursuit of the 'big picture', in this case, to be able to deliver and sustain health improvements and not to become deflected by the 'detail', enabled him to sustain momentum and surmount administrative challenges and hurdles. Inevitably, he relied heavily on a dedicated group of talented thinkers and commissioners at Norad, including the Director Helga Fogstad, Lars Gronseth, Paul Fife and Lene Jeanette Lothe to take care of the detail that fortified the transformational thinking. All of whom witnessed his political tact in accessing people with decision-making power and understanding the systematic process of moving ideas forward and getting policies implemented. To achieve lasting improvements in maternal and child health, Godal knew that he needed access to political influence – this was the realpolitik metric at play in global health. Mostly, he could use his craft and vision working behind the scenes, but on the occasions when direct action was necessary, he was decisive and exercised the power of a trusted emissary. Lene Jeanette Lothe was a colleague of Godal for almost a decade and saw at first hand his ability to bring resources to the table.

> Tore doesn't travel to meetings at the World Bank with big note books; instead he travels with Post-It Notes in his breast pocket. When he was establishing the global campaign for the health MDGs, the prime minister gave him a large chequebook and the flexibility to allocate big sums and to move efforts along. I remember on his Post-It Notes were sums that I had no previous experience of seeing. To create those moments and take decisions he had a lot of trust from the prime minister and I think that he demonstrated that trust led to results. It is an amazing way of working and I don't think we will ever be able to live through it again. It was a one-time experience working with a global leader with a chequebook and the ability to move things around with money.[49]

Godal knew exactly how to prepare the ground, or in the vernacular of global health insider, Suprotik Basu, 'to grease the skids of the UN system', for politicians and decision-makers. In these efforts, he could call upon the dextrous talents of a cadre of high-ranking diplomats including Tarald Brautaset and Morten Wetland. This was vitally important at a time when the gravitational centre of the maternal and child campaign moved to New York City when Ban Ki-moon became Secretary-General of the United Nations in January 2007. The idea was to expand the funding base and get more politically powerful women involved in the Global Campaign for the Health Millennium Development Goals. In 2007, Morten Wetland spoke to a delegation of women from the US congress and harnessing the persuasive power of these influencers became a theme of the maternal and child campaign. A year later, the health MDGs were elevated further up the arc of global politics when Morten Wetland became Norway's new Permanent

Representative to the United Nations, which gave him influence in the form of what he described, 'a key card to the secretary-general's office'.[50]

Every Woman Every Child

In his memoir *A Promised Land*, Barak Obama wrote this intriguing assessment of Ban Ki-moon, the South Korean Secretary-General of the United Nations.

> Two years into his term as the world's most prominent diplomat, Ban Ki-moon had yet to make much of an impression on the global stage. . . . You didn't go into a meeting with Ban expecting to hear captivating stories, witty asides, or dazzling insights. . . . Despite his lack of pizzazz, I would come to like and respect Ban. He was honest, straightforward, and irrepressibly positive. . . . Ban was also persistent.[51]

Ban Ki-moon may have stood in sharp contrast to the erudite charisma of his predecessor at the UN, Kofi Annan, but the two men did have one thing in common, Robert 'Bob' Orr, who served as the United Nations Secretary-General for Policy Cooperation and Strategic Planning, advised them both. In 2007, Bob Orr as head of policy looked around for an issue in the health sphere that would benefit from the new secretary-general's support and leadership. Although the UN secretary-general presides over a large budget, a sprawling bureaucracy and a multitude of international agencies, power is largely dependent on the ability to marshal 193 countries towards something resembling a unifying cause. Therefore, it was incumbent upon Bob Orr to select a campaign for Ban Ki-moon that could transcend national and geopolitical concerns and expand the commitment of the global health assemblage. When Orr sought advice among world experts for an idea that would weave together the technical, political and economic elements of human well-being, one issue immediately came to the fore; women and children's health, and one name persistently came up as being synonymous with the subject, that of Tore Godal. Bob Orr did not have a global health background and had never heard Godal's name before. However, he had worked with many Norwegians during his career at the UN and when he met Godal he recognised the characteristic straightforward demeanour.

> Tore is very plainspoken; step-by-step he outlined his vision to assemble a global health coalition, and he immediately stuck me as an entrepreneur in the space. This was a person quite advanced in his career and he was still thinking like a young-and-coming entrepreneur, 'how can we innovate our way to a better future', that was his mind-set.[52]

The problem Orr faced was that Ban Ki-moon came from a culture in which people are not overtly expressive; consequently, he was reticent and felt deeply uncomfortable talking about his personal history and the tumult of his life as a refugee when his family had to flee from North Korean and Chinese soldiers during the Korean War.[53] Nonetheless, this traumatic, deep-rooted memory had forged an unshakable belief in him that development initiatives must focus on women, but Bob Orr still felt that he needed to expose Ban Ki-moon to a group of global health activists that were passionate, determined and had a workable programme that would improve the health of women and children. To help extricate Ban Ki-moon from his natural hesitancy and persuade him to take a lead on the health of women and children, a gathering of global health leaders took place at the beautiful Greentree estate, a United Nations retreat on Long Island, one hour from Manhattan. The meeting, which was held in a windowless, dark wood panelled room, included such health luminaries as Margaret Chan, Director-General of the WHO, UNICEF leaders, together with leading philanthropic agencies and the subject under discussion was, 'please come and help the UN shape what this agenda for women and children should look like'. Bob Orr drew up the list of attendees, and two of the people he was determined to bring into the discussion were Godal, and Amina Mohammed, who is currently the fifth Deputy Secretary-General of the UN and at the time, was a development entrepreneur working in Nigeria. 'Tore and Amina were my two catalyst instigators who were willing to blow past all of the institutional issues of rivalry that played out at the Greentree meeting: they just had no patience with that'.[54] Godal knew that they had to find a way to overcome internecine squabbles and segregated 'silo' thinking, if he was to put together a unifying world force to improve women and children's health, at a time when ten million children were dying every year,[55] and a pandemic of maternal mortality was sweeping through low-income countries. Bob Orr remembers the absolute intensity of Godal when he explained why a new institutional structure was required. 'Tore told the meeting', remembers Orr,

> the reason why we are not making progress is sitting in this room. We are all looking through different institutional lenses – this is why the secretary-general needs to take a leadership role. Ban Ki-moon is key to getting everyone to work together and get behind this agenda.[56]

Others in the room, including Amina Mohammed, and Agnes Binagwaho, a Rwandan academic and paediatrician, agreed with Godal's sentiments. For too long reducing maternal and childhood mortality had been treated as something of a mythical 'goal' rather than a pledge to invest in the health systems necessary to bring about the 'how' this goal could be realised. Amina Muhammed listed the stark statistics from her country, Nigeria, Africa's most populous nation that had a maternal mortality rate of 1,100 per 100,000. 'That number', Amina Mohammed recounted,

> was just off the scale, and Tore opened up the debate with his salvo. Agnes, myself, and others said, 'cut to the chase', we are not going to finish this

meeting with niceties and going through what we already know. But how are we going to walk out of this room with something that is actually going to make a difference.[57]

There was a feeling that Godal's heartfelt and reasoned appeal evoked in Ban Ki-moon an emotional response that was unexpected in light of his restrained personality, and it had a captivating effect on people. He told a moving story about when he was in a refugee camp as a young child and visited a ramshackle birthing tent with his heavily pregnant mother who was about to give birth to his sister. Standing outside, he watched other pregnant women preparing to enter the tent, and as they did so, they took off their decrepit rubber shoes and looked at them for a very long time. There was an unmistakable plangency to his memory when he recalled the story that his mother had later told him:

> When women were going into labor, they would look at their rubber shoes . . . They would sigh deeply and worry whether they would ever be able to wear those shoes again. I did not understand then what my mother meant. The brutality of childbirth was one thing women could count on in the developing world, including Korea in the 1950s.[58]

The Greentree conference evolved into the *Every Woman Every Child* (EWEC) movement and brought the much-needed political leadership of the UN Secretary-General to a long-neglected health concern. Putting maternal and child health, and survival, at the top of the list of health priorities proved to be a decisive moment in global health. Women and children were *together*, and it gave all the stakeholders an idea of the investments 'needed to give a woman the chance to give birth to a child safely and to survive'.[59] Ban Ki-moon believed sincerely in *Every Woman Every Child*, it was personal for him, and wrote that no single issue ties together the security, prosperity and progress of our world more than women's health.[60] However, the UN is a complex organisation, where myriad campaigns vie for political influence, and in this fractious environment, some fail and atrophy because they do not have the funds, staff or organisation needed to succeed. Godal was determined that this was not going to be the fate of the *Every Woman Every Child* campaign, and he was going to do everything in his power to ensure that, 'by 2010, MDG 4&5 would become the hottest topic in global health'.[61] Using his powerful links in the Norwegian Ministry of Foreign Affairs, Godal secured funding to establish a Secretariat, hosted by the UN Foundation, in effect, a mini-bureaucracy, under the control of Bob Orr that would guide the campaign through the politically congested maze of the United Nations. This action transformed Orr into an empowered civil servant with a line-item budget, a (small) dedicated staff and Ban Ki-moon, the world's most prominent diplomat vowing to use the UN's global infrastructure to make mortality in childbirth 'a rare exception rather than a fatalistic risk'.[62] Now, while there was nothing nefarious about Godal's actions – he was always honest and transparent – and others could have written a cheque if they wished, but no one else had come forward. Intuitively, Godal could sense if momentum was slowing and what was required to move an issue forward.[63] Indeed, as Suprotik Basu has observed, the dynamic had now changed for MDGs 4 and 5:

> the U.N. had now become the bully pulpit, two degrees removed from Tore. He moved quickly, and therefore had influence and *Every Woman Every Child* became real. He knew the political reality of power and influence in these bureaucracies to make things happen. It was ingenious and he could use it to great effect.[64]

Global politics and global health had aligned.

As the first decade of the new millennium was ending, Godal was expanding his commitment to the campaign within the UN system. In 2009, Kathy Calvin was the CEO of the UN foundation, a charitable organisation headquartered in Washington, DC, designed as a strategic partner to the UN for addressing the world's problems. 'Tore recognised that it was his job to mobilise all the rest of us to carry out his vision for EWEC', Kathy Calvin admirably recalled, 'but then made it seem like we owned it!'[65] The CEO soon appreciated that Godal had a deep understanding of how the UN worked and possessed an impressive support network to call upon.

> Tore would say things like, 'if you could deal with Morten and Bob Orr, I think you can make this happen'. Meaning Norway will put some money behind it and Bob will give us approval. Tore was world class and he always kept pushing.[66]

This forward momentum was translating into concrete policies that were making a difference to the health of women and children. First, the debt cancellation that Gordon Brown had orchestrated in the 2005, at the G8 summit at the Gleneagles Hotel, Scotland, had begun to feed into the system. The agreement to write off US\$40 billion owed by the 18 highest indebted countries led to improving health outcomes for maternal health in Nigeria. Amina Mohammed, who was responsible for coordination of Nigeria's debt relief fund and the MDG goals, was able to transform what had been a tragic burden of disease metric.

> I worked with Tore at the UN, and because of the debt relief that we got I was able to put money in and we reduced maternal mortality rates from 1,100 per 100,000 to 550 per 100,000 in a very short space of time.[67]

Second, in January 2010, the Gates Foundation earmarked \$10 billion to kickstart a decade of vaccination in the hope of keeping eight million infants from an early grave from diarrheal disease and pneumonia.[68] Third, the idea of getting more politically powerfully women involved in the *EWEC* movement advanced significantly in terms of resources and convening power with the enthusiastic participation of Melinda Gates. This was a vindication of Bob Orr's attempts to involve all of the non-profit deliverers, the high-finance agencies and the big philanthropists. After the meeting at the Greentree estate, it was Orr's decision to call the new campaign '*Every Woman Every Child*' because he wanted it to reflect something that was universal, ambitious and people centred. The idea was to build a coalition that would bring down institutional barriers and end institutional definitions of health as just a *health* issue. Orr viewed this as a crucial moment in global public health because it brought in a wider constellation of interests.

> With Melinda in the lead on *EWEC* she started to help bring not only the money and the resources of the BMGF but also to bring her vision for looking at women and children's health more integrally and that was of course Consistently what we were trying to do.

Between 2005 and 2010, Godal's vision to question the utility of the whole ecosystem and to bring in new partners had come to fruition. 'Tore was essential in building this coalition', Bob Orr believes, 'and the Norwegian funding was critical because I had nothing, there was nothing in the U.N. for this – so funding and vision were key'.[69] In September 2010, with all the constituent parts in place, Ban Ki-moon officially launched *Every Woman Every Child* as his legacy project at the headquarters of the UN with $40 billion in pledges to reduce maternal and child mortality by 16 million and prevent an estimated 33 million unwanted pregnancies over the next five years.[70] Only five years after Kofi Annan's admonishment of world leaders for not taking the MDGs seriously, the world had been turned upside down, and the political movement to advance maternal and child health according to Godal 'had become the hottest topic in global health!'[71]

In Morten Wetland's long career as a diplomat, he witnessed only two occasions when guests at the UN jettisoned the accepted etiquette of politeness and became belligerent, rough and unruly. Godal, Bob Orr and others had deliberated created a feeling around the *Every Woman Every Child* movement that anyone who truthfully cared about improving the world needed to be at the meeting. Inevitably, this led to the shoehorning of a large and excited crowd into a confined space with understandably combustible consequences. At the time, renovation work was taking place at the UN, and the meeting was held in a temporary building on the north lawn, with the first three rows occupied by presidents, prime ministers and the world's leading philanthropists including Bill and Melinda Gates – the chamber quickly filled to overflowing. To the consternation of Bob Orr, the crush of people in the hallway almost prevented Ban Ki-moon from getting out of the elevator and into the chamber. 'The Fire

Marshall almost shut us down, at no point in the history of the UN had it ever had so many diplomats trying to get into a meeting like this. That was new'. An international breakthrough had taken place based on policy engineering, which enabled the right players to act in unison to do the right thing. Godal knew that for Norway to make a difference at the world level it needed to act strategically, and *Every Woman Every Child* was an important component of his tactical vision to bring the world's focus on this agenda and to align an advocacy campaign to get maternal and child health moving with increasing speed and political weight.

According to the cultural historian, Raymond Williams, each moment in history has its own 'structures of feeling',[72] which change as new things happen and are more widely experienced in a defined period of time. Quite clearly, there was a *feeling* that a decisive point in the history of global health occurred in the summer of 2010, as saving the lives of women and children became the cause that could unite partnerships and mobilise policymakers to move from advocacy to action. Just days after the launch of Ban Ki-moon's legacy project in New York City, the Canadian Prime Minister, Stephen Harper, played host to the 36th G8 summit in Muskoka, Canada on 25–26 June 2010. The annual meeting took place in the aftermath of the greatest economic crisis of modern times and world leaders were looking to address key challenges in environmental protection, international peace and security and development. For 2 days, the Muskoka Summit was the locus of world political power, and in the months leading up to the conference, Tore Godal had been working diligently in Canada advising the office of the prime minister. Harper, like Jens Stoltenberg, was an economist and he admired Norway's commitment to the health MDGs. Making the health MDGs politically thinkable was, according to the Indian-Canadian health economist and epidemiologist, Prabhat Jha, an important factor in Harper's conversion to the ideals of maternal and child health.

> I was involved in the run up to the G8 meeting and getting Stephen Harper to do something serious on maternal and child health. There was a focus on statistics, collecting civil registration, vital statistics, and data investment together with money, ideas, and institutional leadership. No doubt, Tore played a key role in that because he was a Sherpa for the Norwegian government, showing how Canada could punch above its weight in terms of development-assistance, and visited Ottawa in preparation for the launch event in Muskoka (Toronto).[73]

Even in the wake of the global economic meltdown of 2008, there was a discernible shift in the ideological compass of the political leaders at Muskoka – perhaps they were reminded of what the economist John Maynard Keynes wrote during the economic chaos of the World War II: 'Anything we can actually do we can afford'.[74] The appeal of Godal's thinking to politicians was that his programme emphasised the philosophy of the 1993 World Development Report *Investing in*

Health that spending should be on the most cost-effective and measurable interventions that improve outcomes.

Stephen Harper and his wife, Laureen, were highly persuasive hosts and fully embraced the idea of making progress on reducing child mortality and 'the need to support mothers both at home and abroad'. At the end of the G8 Summit, Harper launched the *Muskoka Initiative*, a comprehensive and integrated approach to accelerate progress towards MDGs 4 and 5 aimed at significantly reducing the number of maternal, newborn and under-five child death in developing countries. Moreover, this huge step forward in ending avoidable mortality was more than a noble ambition, with $5 billion in additional funding from the rich G8 countries over five years. The undertaking aimed to support and strengthen country-led national health systems in developing countries in sustainable ways.[75] This support from the G8 was synergistic; and a collective effort from the governments of Holland, New Zealand, Norway, the Republic of Korea, Spain, Switzerland and the Bill and Melinda Gates Foundation led to another $5 billion in funding over the same period. What was particularly satisfying for Godal was that the four biggest NGOs contributed even more financial support than the world's richest industrial nations. The *Muskoka Initiative* added momentum to the UN-led *Joint Action Plan to Improve the Health of Women and Children* that was to take centre stage at the prestigious UN Plenary Meeting in September 2010, in New York City.

The UN Commission on Life-Saving Commodities for Women and Children

The political influence generated over the summer for maternal and child health gained further traction within the media through a highly effective public relations effort orchestrated by Marshall Hoffman, an astute US campaigner, who had worked closely with Godal at the WHO in the 1980s. Hoffman could be unorthodox, even brash, and he upset people in the communication divisions of organisations because he wanted to work directly with experts, but Godal liked Hoffmann because 'he delivers'.[76] Hoffman's global media outreach strategy was to create a sense of purposeful excitement around the subject. This led to a highly effective campaign that included an avalanche of tactically deployed press releases in national newspapers and on radio and television, together with promotional videos that featured among others, the Hollywood actor Jennifer Lopez and the international best-selling singer, Celine Dion, in support of maternal and child health. This media campaign was indispensable and helped to mobilise political support in the United States and beyond.

Furthermore, by the late summer of 2010, the vaccination programmes that Godal had overseen at GAVI, combined with the protective effects of insecticide-treated bed nets in areas of high malaria transmission which he had implemented in his TDR career, began to feed through in the form of reduced levels of mortality. These life-saving innovations led the UN Secretary-General to invite Godal to head a working group on innovation in health services for women and children. Uncharacteristically, because of his customary reticence, Godal's contribution of global public health appeared on the front page of the *New York Times*. Morten Wetland wanted to strike a historical chord when describing Godal's commitment to human well-being.

> Because the Norwegian polar explorer and diplomat, Fridtjof Nansen[77] had saved so many lives in the twentieth century, we wanted to draw parallels between their shared contributions, and we managed to get it on the front page of the *New York Times*.[78]

Jens Stoltenberg reinforced this historical lineage by declaring, 'Dr Godal's efforts to improve the health of the poor are inestimable. After Fridtjof Nansen, he is probably the Norwegian whose work has saved the most lives'.[79] This eminence was contradictory, because while Godal cares deeply about the impact and the results, he is little interested in the vanity around it. However, in the environment of high-stakes politics he was peerless. His modesty, and efforts to remain undetectable in the limelight, was accompanied by a self-assurance that assuaged any misgivings that potential partners may have had. According to his WHO colleague and friend, David Nabarro, 'Tore has self-confidence from the bottom of his toes to the top of his head'. As an experienced public servant, he had learnt a valuable lesson that it is often possible to do more by saying less. In this sense, he followed the beliefs of the medieval philosopher William of Occam, and his 'principles of parsimony' (Occam's Razor) that made the world simpler and more comprehensible.[80] Crucially, Godal had a talent to simplify complexity for politicians and condense things down to a few memorable sentences or 'action points' and 'next steps'.[81] Quite simply, he spoke their language and, in turn, made politicians shine: this enabled Stoltenberg and him to put together a global network made up of 11 heads of state, health ministers and other decision-makers that became the motor driving improved health services for the world's poorest women and children.[82] There is little doubt that the network of global leaders moulded by Godal and Prime Minister Stoltenberg was catalytic. 'Soon afterwards', Godal told a medical journal, 'our discussions were being presented at the UN General Assembly and the world started to take notice'.[83]

In September 2010, Ban Ki-moon's global strategy for women and children's health highlighted the suffering causes by the lack of access to life-saving commodities. This stark exposure of unmet clinical need came from research carried out by Godal, and his dedicated, close-knit Norad (The Norwegian Agency for Development Cooperation) team, which suggested that the widespread availability of essential life-saving commodities had the power to save millions of lives in low-income countries. Their powerful cause-and-effect analysis led directly to the establishment of the UN Commission on Life-Saving Commodities for

Women and Children, jointly chaired by Goodluck Ebele Jonathan President of Nigeria, and Jens Stoltenberg, Prime Minister of Norway.[84] When the Commission reported two years later, its findings were unequivocal. It identified '13 overlooked life-saving commodities that if more widely accessed and properly used, could save the lives of more than 6 million women and children'.[85] The Commission's recommendations identified excessive bleeding as the most dangerous and substantial complication of giving birth, and pneumonia and diarrhoeal diseases as causing greatest mortality in early life.

The 13 commodities and the medical conditions they prevent:

- Oxytocin (postpartum haemorrhage)
- Misoprostol (postpartum haemorrhage)
- Magnesium sulphate (eclampsia and sever pre-eclampsia)
- Injectable antibiotics (newborn sepsis)
- Antenatal corticosteroids – ANCs (preterm respiratory distress syndrome)
- Chlorhexidine (newborn cord care)
- Resuscitation devices (newborn asphyxia)
- Amoxicillin (pneumonia)
- Oral rehydration salts – ORS (diarrhoea)
- Zinc (diarrhoeas)
- Female condoms (family planning and contraception)
- Contraceptive implants (family planning and contraception)
- Emergency contraception (family planning and contraception)

The Commission's strategy called on the global community to work together to save 16 million lives by 2015, and effectively address avoidable causes of death during pregnancy, childbirth and childhood. To achieve the objective, the Commission listed ten recommendations and called for 'innovative financing' to address the economic barriers to ensure that the poorest members of society have access to the life-saving commodities. In support of the commission's report, the *Global Campaign for the Health MDGs* launched its report *Accelerating progress in saving the lives of Women and Children*. Godal oversaw the contents and cadence of the report, ably assisted by his Norad colleagues. Global health appeared to had moved into a new era, moving past the stage of development assistance to country ownership and global cooperation. Furthermore, Godal strengthened the reverberating Brownian motion of creativity and innovation that represented the transformed 'structures of feeling' surrounding the MDGs 4 and 5 with a series of collaborative articles in *The Lancet* as the 2015 MDG deadline approached.[86] This contributed to what Suprotik Basu succinctly termed, 'a wonderful five-year sweet spot for the MDGs 4&5. Because 31 December 2015 was close enough so that it got people nervous, but far enough away that we could still get some work done'.[87] On 19 May 2014, Tore Godal's 75th birthday was celebrated in a profile article written by his friend, and Head of Health at

Norad, Helga Fogstad, which catalogued his lasting contributions to global public health. 'Since the MDGs started', Fogstad wrote, '6.5 million children are saved every year from dying'.[88] In 2005, Godal had initiated an evidence-based campaign aimed at improving child and maternal health, and within a decade, unprecedented improvements in rates of preventable deaths had been made. However, his 75th birthday did not signal any slowdown in his push for greater and sustainable progress. 'A million more', Godal said, 'and we will reach the Millennium Development Goal, however, this is not enough. There are still four million dying from diseases that can be prevented'. Yet a historic milestone was about to be reached. Between 2010 and 2015, the progress in child and maternal health was the fastest ever recorded. With global under-five mortality rates declining by over 50% since 1990, while global maternal death rates dropped by almost 40% in the same period.

During Godal's ten-year campaign, the hallmarks of his work were tireless persistence and attention to detail, operational qualities that would serve him well in his efforts to persuade the hierarchy of the World Bank, to introduce a new system of innovative financing to ensure that the advances in maternal and child health would be sustainable and permanent. With the MDGs due to be superseded in 2015 by the Sustainable Development Goals – a collection of 17 interrelated objectives selected by the UN General Assembly – Godal was determined to align the *Every Woman Every Child* ethos into this new global health architecture, and he wanted to be directly involved. However, he was also a clear-eyed realist, and he knew that to fashion a relationship with the World Bank, and directly influence the institution's development ideology, his best opportunity would come when the conservative-minded, fiscally prudent UN agency was in a state of flux. Just such an opportunity arose in May 2014 when the Canadian government held the maternal and child health conference *Saving Every Woman and Every Child* seeking to galvanise support for the next phase of efforts and ensure that maternal, newborn and child health continued to be a global priority. Among the high-level speakers, attending the 3-day conference was Ban Ki-moon, and the Korean born, US president of the World Bank president, Jim Yong Kim. Jim Kim was an anomaly in the history of the World Bank, because as well as being the first president not to have a background in the political or financial sector, he was a medic, with a career in global health. At a breakfast gathering on the first morning of the conference, the delegates shared a genuine sense of camaraderie and a personalised connection to the issue of maternal health – the Tanzanian President Jakaya Kikwete's mother died in childbirth – infused the room. Jim Kim was also 'excited'[89] about the subject and wanted to do more to end preventable deaths and launch an inventive financial modality to transfer World Bank resources to cost-effective interventions. This heightened sense of purpose led Jim Kim to make his pitch and declare to the other global health leaders that the World Bank would, under his stewardship, expand its financial commitment to match the demands of developing countries' needs to improve maternal and child health care. In a brilliant exposition, Richard Horton eloquently describes how Jim Kim's breakfast declaration, while well-meaning, went beyond his remit, and contravened one of the Bank's unwritten guiding principles, and in so doing gave Tore Godal the opportunity he was looking for to influence and increase the flow of resources to MDGs 4 and 5.

> When Jim Kim made the promise that the World Bank was going to give a shedload of money, the problem was he hadn't got it in his power to give money. Funds could not be earmarked for women and children's health, so they had to concoct a mechanism by which the World Bank could save face and provide a financing mechanism. And Ariel Pablos-Mendez at The United States Agency for International Aid (USAID), and Tim Evans at the World Bank together with Tore concocted the Global Financing Facility to dig the Bank out of a hole.[90]

This trenchant synopsis of the unforeseen consequences of Jim Kim's breakfast speech did indeed necessitate the fabrication of an entirely novel system of innovative financing at the World Bank and ushered in a new era of results-based financing that placed Godal at the centre of a panoramic vision for global health.

The Global Financing Facility

When the Health Innovation Trust Fund was established at the World Bank in 2007, it linked the Norwegian investment in results-based finance to the International Development Association (IDA), the concessional loans or grant for low-income countries from the Bank.[91] Initially, Godal had been concerned that this linkage would overtly bureaucratise the funding process but was willing to go along with the experiment because Amie Batson told him that IDA and its potential excited World Bank staff. The Health Innovation Trust Fund grew slowly and the managers were, to Godal's mind, of varying quality until Monique Vledder took control in 2012. Vledder, a young, decisive and visionary thinker inherited a mechanism that had a lot of money but very few projects to finance. Now with the guiding roadmap discoveries of the Commission on Life-Saving Commodities, and the commitment made by Jim Kim, Vledder and Tim Evans, Director of Health, Nutrition and Population at the World Bank, decided to 'convert the Health Innovation Trust Fund into a new entity, the Global Financing Facility',[92] and link investments in the health sector to better outcomes for women and children. To ensure that the new venture had a successful presentation at the UN General Assembly in late September 2014, Godal knew that he would need to persuade Norway's politicians to make an even greater contribution to long-term global health spending. Such an undertaking would have been difficult to secure at any time; however, in 2013 the political status quo had been dramatically recalibrated, when Jens Stoltenberg's Labour Party lost the general election on

9 September, and Erna Solberg was elected prime minister of a right-of-centre government. In late August 2014, and with the all-important UN General Assembly meeting only a matter of days away, Godal attended a meeting in the Ministry of Foreign Affairs, with a Deputy State Secretary – their conversation centred around the delicate issue of how to get the anti-aid populist progressive party on board for a global health aid programme! However, when Godal introduced the idea of results-based financing the Deputy State Secretary became 'very enthusiastic',[93] principally because Erna Solberg was an extremely skilful politician and engaged with public health issues, having a particular interest in gender issues and education.[94] In this sense, the Prime Minister viewed health and education as two sides of the same coin; seeing that attending school but not being immunised was detrimental to a child's health. Likewise, being vaccinated against infectious diseases but having no access to education was equally disadvantageous. Marshall Hoffmann once wrote that 'Tore Godal takes big chances',[95] and it was certainly true that Godal and his global public health policies were ideologically linked with Jens Stoltenberg and the Labour Party which had dominated Norwegian political and cultural life for most of the previous decade. Nevertheless, by advocating a policy that was 'results focused', Godal successfully transcended the political divide and managed to persuade Erna Solberg, and her new government, to wholeheartedly support the Global Financing Facility and its ideals of equity, transparency and cost-effectiveness. At the end of September 2014, Erna Solberg endorsed the concept of the Global Financing Facility at the United Nations General Assembly while sharing a platform with the United Nation's Secretary-General Ban Ki-moon, World Bank President, Jim Kim and the Canadian Prime Minister Stephen Harper. In doing so, she announced a doubling of the Norwegian contribution to $600 million for six years. Far from being ideologically reluctant to spend large sums on development aid, Norway made the first pledge to the GFF, and Canada immediately followed with a donation of $200 million, making the combined sum, $800 million. The political allegiance of successive Norwegian prime ministers to the ideals of the health MDGs, which began with a global campaign in 2007, was now complete.[96]

Throughout the hectic months leading up to the announcement of the GFF in 2014, Monique Vledder worked closely with Godal and came to admire his intellectual horsepower, perseverance and sheer ubiquity. Regardless of whether a global health conference was taking place in Accra, Djibouti or Kyoto, there was an inescapable feeling that a worldwide network of global health experts existed in which *Tore Godal knew everyone and everyone in turn knew Tore Godal*. 'I have this image of him', Monique Vledder remembered with amusement,

in bright yellow sneakers at the World Health Assembly, or in bright blue sneakers, at the United Nations General Assembly, and he would spend the entire week walking from one coffee to another, because everyone would be in town. And he has a plan, a direction – and he was already well into his seventies by then. It is incredible what he can do. He is so incredibly disciplined, and I think he can do it, because he truly deeply cares. It is a life-dedication.[97]

It has never been easy or straightforward, to raise funds for women and children's health, and in the months leading up to the September meeting in New York City Godal had to delicately manoeuvre politicians, the hierarchy of the World Bank Group and international aid agencies to create the Global Financing Facility. This was a game of high-stakes poker, which took Godal, and Helga Fogstad, across the world and into the citadels of financial and political power in the United Kingdom, the United States, across the continent of Europe and beyond. 'Deals were made', Helga Fogstad remembers, 'that no-one else could have possibly brokered because of Tore's powers of persuasion and credibility'.[98] In playing a form of high-stakes poker to secure funding for some the world's most disadvantaged people, Godal followed the allegorical advice of the 1970s country music song 'The Gambler', *You never count your money, When you're sittin' at the table*, and if the dramatic breakthrough was to be achieved then, *You've got to know when to hold 'em, Know when to fold 'em.* . . . In the opinion of Monique Vledder, it was Godal's inventive daring, and impeccable sense of timing, that brought a theatrical flourish to the UN General Assembly meeting in New York.

> At that moment in September, Tore had to twist himself in all kinds of ways to pool that money from different sources, but he knew – and again, this is the politician in him – that people would only start paying attention if there was a big number. If you try to establish something new with $50 million, nothing will happen, but with $800 million! We could then agree that the World Bank would connect the IDA funding, leveraging about $5 billion in the initial phase.[99]

The metrics of this umbilical arrangement were compelling. For every dollar invested by Norway, IDA put in four or five dollars (rising to seven dollars by 2021). As a direct consequence of linking the funding from donors like Norway, to the IDA, it led to very substantial increases in funding from IDA for maternal and child health. However, brokering this arrangement was extremely complex and tested the philosophical principles that guided the World Bank's investment strategy since its inception in 1944.

The International Development Association (IDA) is the part of the World Bank that helps the world's poorest countries by providing zero or low-interest loans, grants or 'credits' for programmes to reduce poverty, boost economic growth and improve people's living standards. What Monique Vledder and Godal envisioned was to position health at the centre of development; this was to be achieved by strengthening health systems at the country level, allowing each individual country to make their own decisions and build from the bottom-up an integrated maternal and child health service. This vision for the health MDGs and earmarking funds for specific health outcome did not sit well, as Jim Kim found out, with the economic theologians at the World Bank. Suprotik Basu and Monique Vledder joined the World Bank within a few days of each other at the beginning of this century, and Basu was keenly aware of the opposition that existed within the Bank to the GFF ideal.

> 'Earmarking', within the Bank is such a dirty word, and many of the IDA deputies hated the idea. . . . Obviously, the Covid-pandemic has put health at the centre of development. But at the time, the Bank put up all sorts of reasons why countries don't borrow for *health*. The Bank wanted to loan money for infrastructure and hard assets and the economists and engineers made it very difficult for the Health Ministries to access funding. Tore knew this, and by combining a 'loan' and a 'grant', it worked as an incentive, because countries knew that if they could take IDA for maternal and child health they would also get the grant funding which would mitigate much of the cost. This was free cash, and free cash leads you to the Finance Ministers doors. And I think some people considered Tore to be unfairly putting his thumb on the scales to unlock the World Bank's money, when he shouldn't have unlocked it in that way.[100]

Historically, the Health Ministries in developing countries had been at the bottom of the totem pole power structure, and Godal was determined to provide a mechanism that gave health the purchasing power to pursue policies that would reduce poverty, aid development and improve health outcomes. To achieve this, he needed the convening power and political muscle of Ariel Pablos-Mendez, who led the Global Health Bureau of USAID, and was leader of End Premature Child and Maternal Death in the government of President Barak Obama.

By his own admission, Ariel Pablos-Mendez began his career in global health 'by accident'[101] in the 1990s, when as a physician, he began investigating multi-drug-resistant tuberculosis within New York City's homeless population. He went on to work at the Rockefeller Foundation with his friend and colleague, Tim Evans, where he developed a portfolio of drugs and vaccines for the diseases of the poor. This concentration on the neglected diseases of poverty in turn brought him into contact with Godal, Director of TDR at the end of the last century when both were influential members of a Working Group that became the Medicines for Malaria Venture (MMV). In the first decade of the new millennium, Pablos-Mendez shepherded the Rockefeller Foundation's initiative on the transformation of health systems towards universal health coverage, before becoming Head of Maternal and Child Health at USAID. This was in the aftermath of the great economic recession of 2008, and the collapse of the financial markets made it essential to invent a new mechanism for development assistance for health at the country level. Clearly, the exponential growth in global health spending that had reached over US$30 billion a year was coming to an end,[102] and as Pablos-Mendez found out, even USAID, the world's largest aid agency, was not immune to the new realities.

> I tried to make a case for the reduction of child mortality in the National Security Council. This was when we were investing four times as many dollars on HIV/AIDS than in child mortality even though we had four times as many child deaths than deaths from the AIDS epidemic. But I couldn't get a big new check![103]

This was the historical context to the unfolding impasse confronting global health strategists during the summer of 2014. On the one hand, the GFF was an attempt to do things in a new way, in response to the new economic realities, while on the other, its creation, design and eventual success was brought about by old friendships, and a shared vision for maternal and child health.

In June 2014, Ariel Pablos-Mendez and Tim Evans shared an apartment in Washington, DC. Evans had recently returned from working in Bangladesh and was busy looking for a house for his family to be able to join him in the US capitol; meanwhile, Pablos-Mendez communed back to his family at weekends in New York City where his children were at school. Sharing an apartment gave the two global health experts time to brainstorm about how best to provide essential health services in a time of economic austerity. With many emerging economies growing rapidly, they felt that salvation lay in local resources, country ownership and global cooperation. 'I believed that the new initiative', Ariel Pablos-Mendez wrote in his diary,

> should have more local capacity, more local leadership, and more local resources. At the beginning of June, I laid down a vision for a Global Fund for Maternal and Child Health linking it to the one area of finance that was growing – the IDA loans at the World Bank. I got the idea because we needed to do something different.[104]

Godal, Evans and Pablos-Mendez all wanted the countries to be in charge in the new system and not be *directed* from the North with the accompanying loud echoes of European colonialism. On 25 June, Ariel Pablos-Mendez convened a meeting at USAID attended by Jim Kim, Chris Elias, a senior figure at the Bill and Melinda Gates Foundation, Tim Evans and Tore Godal. Underplaying his part in the meeting, Pablos-Mendez referred to his role as 'just a pot-stirrer', but together they had succeeded in getting Jim Kim, the president of the World Bank, 'on board' and he felt confident enough 'to inform the White House' about a new idea that could reshape global health finance.[105]

Some of the interactions involving the GFF were demanding and complex, for example, the Republican controlled Congress did not like giving money to the

World Bank, and abundant and complex game theory was applied to get things up and running. Nonetheless, rather than mathematic models of strategic inter-action, the decisive element in the GFF story was the strong bond of friendship between the central characters which, in turn, shaped a wider consensus between Norway, USAID and the World Bank. On 26 June, at the Headquarters of the World Bank, in Washington, DC, Tore Godal, Tim Evans and Ariel Pablos-Mendez were called to a meeting in Jim Kim's office. 'On that day', Pablos-Mendez wrote in his diary entry,

> I could see the power of ideas to change the world. The idea clicked in Jim Kim's mind, and he agreed. Of course, I knew him very well, because he had started his career in drug-resistant tuberculosis in Peru. He was my friend and he trusted me. Looking back we were like the Three Musketeers: Tore repre-senting Norway, Tim the World Bank, and me USAID. After the meeting, the three of us went back to Tim's office. We were really happy and celebrated with a cold beer![106]

Throughout the summer of 2014, Godal had been indefatigable in his efforts to build a call to action across the world assemblage to address the maternal and child health challenges. As a result, member state organisations like the World Bank and WHO – together with other public and private entities – combined, enabling the Global Finance Facility to become a central actor in the field of health finance. Consequently, it seemed only fitting that the GFF was officially launched in 2015, at the Third International Conference on Financing for Devel-opment, held in Addis Ababa, Ethiopia, which positioned domestic resource allocation at the heart of the post-2015 agenda.[107] In 2018, Norway together with more than 10 other investor nations, including Canada, Germany and France together with The Gates Foundation and the GFF catalysed close financial mech-anisms with The Global Fund and GAVI. For those trying to assemble a new world health era after the Great Recession of 2008, it seemed that with the crea-tion of the GFF, the future had arrived.

In examining the role of the health MDGs, no one can doubt the unprecedented achievements that have been made; between 1990 (the baseline for the MDGs) and 2015, child and maternal deaths decreased by around 50%. This great ben-efit for human health was in the view of Richard Horton easily explained in the context of the difficult art, science and politics of setting cost-effective health priorities in a systematic manner.

> Back in the early MDG era nobody was paying any attention to MDGs 4&5, it was all about AIDS, which is fine, but 4 and 5 were completely ignored. And what Tore did was, and this is why Norway is so fascinating, they chose a subject that was completely ignored by everybody else, and they put in substantial amounts of money. The only reason Norway did that was because

Tore had persuaded Jens Stoltenberg that they could make a difference. That was a journey that Stoltenberg took as prime minister with Tore literally sitting on his shoulder advising him the whole way through. All of us in global health admired that, and it was an astonishing success.[108]

Providing strategic direction was Godal's forte not only in Norway but also in the global context too according to Amina Mohammed who was the touchstone in health.

In his very unassuming way he would give you steel in your spine to go out and do what you had to do. We trusted him. When it came to the Global Financing Facility that the World Bank anchored, he was a big part of that, because he had a reputation for setting up [trust] funds. He brought the weight of Norway behind him and that brought integrity, not because of Norway, but because of him![109]

It was Godal's concern for the vulnerability of people who didn't have health care that was to prove a decisive factor, and his work is an affirmation that as a global society we can do things better. In the Venn diagram intersection, the purple in the middle of the red and blue circles is where Suprotik Basu sees Godal's telling contribution,

the overlap is his effectiveness and his humility and his ability to put the work first. This attracts people to his causes because they know he is not furthering his brand, or ego. . . . Everyone knew Tore was the quiet guy in the corner but probably the one pulling all of the strings.[110]

Norway stands as an exemplar of how a small country can have a big role on the world stage, and the financial resources that Norway can bring to the global table were matched by the quality of the country's human resources and the values they represented. Bob Orr saw these values and social mores were indicative of Godal's leadership style, 'Tore, whipped his own government into shape on maternal and child health and showed how a small country could play a global role and he brought the whole Norwegian government with him'.[111] In 2019, on Tore Godal's 80th birthday, his friend and NATO Secretary-General Jens Stoltenberg sent birthday wishes via a video link from the NATO Headquarters in Brussels and made a joke about Godal being the most expensive Norwegian in history. Later that year, he put his statement into context.

Tore convinced me, the parliament, government, the whole of Norway that we should become the lead nation for child health and vaccines. Thanks to Tore's work, millions of children have become inoculated and child mortality has dropped. No one else could have convinced me to spend billions on child health and maternal care. The money has been very well spent.[112]

One person who understands the power and role of money in global health politics is Monique Vledder, Head of the Global Financing Facility.

Tore is incredibly sophisticated technically, and he has the relationships and access to the political level. And what Tore wants he usually gets, so it is really fortunate for the world that what Tore usually wants is beneficial for other people.[113]

Tore Godal believes we should never accept inequalities in the chances of child survival. One of his early allies in the global campaign against global poverty is Gordon Brown, the former UK prime minister. In his latest book on how to rebuild a world, that is greener, cleaner and fairer, he illustrates just how much work there is still to do.

Most people would rightly regard as morally abhorrent the proposition that a child born into the poorest 20 per cent of a population should face a risk of mortality twice as high as a child born into the richest 20 per cent. Yet that is the reality of the world we now live in.[114]

Notes

1. Interview with Jens Stoltenberg, April 2019.
2. K. Warren, "The difficult art, science, and politics of setting health priorities", *Lancet*, 27 August 1988, pp. 498–499.
3. The Millennium Development Goals set a target for human development for 2015 (against a 1990 baseline).
4. Interview with Jens Stoltenberg, April 2019.
5. S. Boseley, "Norway's Prime Minister Jens Stoltenberg: Leader on MDG 4", *Lancet*, 22 September 2007, 340 (9592), p. 1027.
6. Stoltenberg was born, in 1959, into a leading Norwegian political family – his father, Thorvald Stoltenberg, was a former Foreign Minister.
7. Interview with Richard Horton, August 2020.
8. Interview with Kathy Calvin, June 2021.
9. Interview with Jens Stoltenberg, April 2019.
10. www.fhi.no/en/news/2019/tore-godal-kings-medal-of-merit/ (accessed on 9 October 2021).
11. P. B. Medawar, *The Art of the Soluble: Creating and Originality in Science* (London: Methuen, 1967).
12. T. Godal, "Targeting the health MDGs", *Finance and Development, IMF*, 2007, 0044 (044), p. 38.
13. Interview with Jens Stoltenberg, April 2019.
14. At the end of 2005, when Stoltenberg became Prime Minister, he resigned from the GAVI board after attending one meeting in India.

15. Interview with Richard Horton, August 2020.
16. Interview with Monique Vledder, May 2021.
17. Interview with Jonas Ghar Støre, March 2019.
18. Interview with Bard Vegar Solhjell, July 2021.
19. Interview with Morten Wetland, June 2021.
20. Helga Fogstad speech at Ann Kern-Godal's memorial service, 2 June 2017.
21. Interview with Jens Stoltenberg, April 2019.
22. Interview with Bard Vegar Solhjell, July 2021.
23. Interview with Jens Stoltenberg, April 2019.
24. Interview with Suprotik Basu, July 2021.
25. Interview with Morten Wetland, June 2021.
26. Interview with Richard Horton, August 2020.
27. Interview with Suprotik Basu, July 2021.
28. T. Godal, "Targeting the health MDGs", (in Is the Global Health System Broken?), *Finance & Development, International Monetary Fund*, 2007, p. 38.
29. Interview with Tore Godal, August 2018.
30. T. Godal, "Targeting the health MDGs", (in Is the Global Health System Broken?), *Finance & Development, International Monetary Fund*, 2007, p. 38.
31. Interview with Helga Fogstad, June 2020.
32. S. Boseley, "Norway's Prime Minister Jens Stoltenberg: Leader on MDG 4", *Lancet*, 22 September 2007, 340 (9592), p. 1027.
33. Interview with Morten Wetland, June 2021.
34. T. Godal, "Targeting the health MDGs", (in Is the Global Health System Broken?), *Finance & Development, International Monetary Fund*, 2007, p. 38.
35. Interview with Jens Stoltenberg, April 2019.
36. Interview with Tore Godal, August 2018.
37. NIPI's impact has been impressive. The Government of India has scaled up ten of 11 NIPI innovations. NIPI provision has cared for more than 700,000 newborn and infants and over 5,000 mothers. Since 2006, NIPI has trained over 40,000 health workers. Moreover, and impressive sustainable mechanism has been established – for every Norwegian Kroner (NOK) invested by NIPI, the Government of India invested NOK 19.50 from the state health funds for NIPI innovations.
38. Personal communication, email Rannveig Rajendram, July 2021.
39. Interview with Bård Vegar Solhjell, July 2021.
40. World Health Organization, *World Health Report 2005: Make Every Mother and Child Count* (Geneva: World Health Organization, 2005).
41. G. Jones, R. Steketee, R. E. Black, Z. A. Bhutto, S. S. Morris, Bellagio Child Survival Study Group, "How many child deaths can we prevent this year?", *Lancet*, 2003, 362 (9377), pp. 65–71.
42. G. Brown, *Seven Ways to Change the World: How to Fix the Most Pressing Problems We Face* (London: Simon & Schuster, 2021).
43. Interview with Morten Wetland, June 2021.
44. S. Boseley, "Norway's Prime Minister Jens Stoltenberg: Leader on MDG 4", *Lancet*, 22 September 2007, 340 (9592), p. 1027.
45. Editorial, "International health partnerships: A welcome initiative", *Lancet*, 8 September 2007, 370 (9590), p. 801.
46. T. Godal, "Targeting the health MDGs'", (in Is the Global Health System Broken?), *Finance & Development, International Monetary Fund*, 2007, p. 38.
47. The US chemist and inventor, Spencer Silver, invented the Post-It Note. In 1968, while working at 3M, Silver created a unique adhesive that brought the Post-it Note into being. He promoted his adhesive so tirelessly that he became known as 'Mr

Persistent'. The breakthrough came when a colleague saw a use for the light adhesive to anchor a bookmark in his hymnbook.

48. R. Shah, "Breakthroughs for development", *Science*, 22 July 2011, 333 (6041), p. 385.
49. Interview with Lene Jeanette Lothe, April 2020.
50. Interview with Morten Wetland, June 2021.
51. B. Obama, *A Promised Land* (New York: Viking, 2020), pp. 508–509.
52. Interview with Robert Orr, July 2021.
53. B. Ki-moon, *Resolved Uniting Nations in a Divided World* (New York: Columbia University Press, 2021), p. 238.
54. Interview with Robert Orr, July 2021.
55. R. E. Black, S. S. Morris, J. Bryce, "Where and why are 10 million children dying every year?", *Lancet*, 2003, 361, pp. 2226–2234.
56. Interview with Robert Orr, July 2021.
57. Interview with Amina Mohammed, August 2021.
58. B. Ki-moon, *Resolved Uniting Nations in a Divided World* (New York: Columbia University 2021), p. 250.
59. Interview with Amina Mohammed, August 2021.
60. B. Ki-moon, *Resolved Uniting Nations in a Divided World* (New York: Columbia University Press, 2021), p. 243.
61. Interview with Tore Godal, November 2019.
62. B. Ki-moon, *Resolved Uniting Nations in a Divided World* (New York: Columbia University Press, 2021), p. 243.
63. Interview with Kathy Calvin, July 2021.
64. Interview with Suprotik Basu, July 2021.
65. Interview with Kathy Calvin, July 2021.
66. Interview with Kathy Calvin, July 2021.
67. Interview with Amina Muhammed, August 2021.
68. *The Guardian*, leader article, "In praise of long-life vaccines", 19 February 2010.
69. Interview with Robert Orr, July 2021.
70. B. Ki-moon, *Resolved Uniting Nations in a Divided World* (New York: Columbia University Press, 2021), p. 243.
71. Interview with Tore Godal, November 2019.
72. R. Williams, *Marxism and Literature* (Oxford: Oxford University Press, 1977), p. 128.
73. Interview with Prabhat Jha, February 2020.
74. A. Pettifor, "'Deficit financing' or 'deficit-reduction financing?' Debates in contemporary economics: Origins, confusions and clarity", *Journal of King Abdulaziz University: Islamic Economics*, January 2019, 32 (1), p. 74.
75. The Muskoka Summit took place two-thirds the way through the life of the Millennium Development Goals, which set a target for human development for 2015 (against a 1990 baseline).
76. Interview with Tore Godal, September 2021.
77. A 1920 conference of the League of Nations began the process of agreeing international standards for passports and ensuring any citizen could have one for a reasonable fee. The League issued 'Nansen' passports, informally named after their promoter, the polar explorer Fridtjof Nansen, in the 1920s. They were given to refugees after the chaos of World War I and the Russian revolution. Nansen passports enabled, rather than restricted, the freedoms of those refugees. The passports saved their lives. The Nansen International Office for Refugees received the Nobel Peace Prize in 1930.
78. Interview with Morten Wetland, June 2021.

79. Interview with Jens Stoltenberg, April 2019.

80. Occam's Razor is a set of principles, astonishing in its simplicity, that states it is futile to do with more what can be done with less. In Occam's logic, the only way to gain sure knowledge is through experience and observation, what we would term today as trial and error, which forms the cornerstone of modern science.

81. Interview with Lars Gronseth, September 2021.

82. The other leaders were President Michelle Bachelet of Chile, Prime Minister Jan Peter Balkenende of the Netherlands, Prime Minister Gordon Brown of the United Kingdom, President Armando Guebuza of Mozambique, President Jakaya Kikwete of Tanzania, Prime Minister Kevin Rudd of Australia, President Luiz Inácio Lula da Silva of Brazil, President Ellen Johnson Sirleaf of Liberia, President Abdoulaye Wade of Senegal, President Susilo Bambang Yudhoyono of Indonesia, and Graça Machel, President and founder, Foundation for Community Development Mozambique.

83. R. Lane, "Profile: Tore Godal: Quiet colossus of global health", *Lancet*, 14 December 2019, 394 (10215), p. 2142.

84. *Leading by Example – Protecting the most vulnerable during the economic crisis: The Global Campaign for the Health Millennium Development Goals 2009*, Published by the Office of the Prime Minister of Norway, Oslo, June, 2009. (Printed by Møklegaards Trykkeri AS).

85. *UN Commission on Life-Saving Commodities for Women and Children*, Commissioners' Report, September 2012 (New York), p. 2.

86. T. Godal, R. Klausner, "Innovating for every woman and every child", *Lancet*, 2012, 379 (9810), pp. el–e2.

    T. Godal, L. Quam, "Accelerating the global response to reduce maternal mortality", *Lancet*, 2 June 2012, 379 (9831), pp. 2025–2026.

    S. Berkley, M. Dybul, T. Godal, A. Lake, "Integration and innovation to advance newborn survival", *Lancet*, 2014, 384 (9938), pp. e22–e23.

87. Interview with Suprotik Basu, July 2021.

88. R. Lane, "Profile: Tore Godal: Quiet colossus of global health", *Lancet*, 14 December 2019, 394 (10215), p. 2142.

89. Interview with Monique Vledder, May 2021.

90. Interview with Richard Horton, August 2020.

91. The International Development Association (IDA) is the part of the World Bank that helps the world's poorest countries. Overseen by 173 shareholder nations, IDA aims to reduce poverty by providing zero to low-interest loans (called 'credits') and grants for programs that boost economic growth, reduce inequalities and improve people's living conditions.

92. Interview with Monique Vledder, May 2021.

93. Interview with Tore Godal, August 2018.

94. Interview with Bard Vegar Solhjell, July 2021.

95. Email communication with Marshall Hoffmann, September 2021.

96. In 2013, Erna Solberg became an MDG Advocate and in 2016 co-chaired the UN Secretary General's Advocacy group of Sustainable Development Goals.

97. Interview with Monique Vledder, May 2021.

98. Interview with Helga Fogstad, June 2020.

99. Interview with Monique Vledder, May 2021.

100. Interview with Suprotik Basu, July 2021.

101. Interview with Ariel Pablos-Mendez, May 2020.

102. A. Pablos-Mendez, M. C. Raviglione, "A new world health era", *Global Health: Science and Practice*, 21 March 2018, 6 (1), p. 1.

103. Interview with Ariel Pablos-Mendez, May 2020.
104. Interview with Ariel Pablos-Mendez, May 2020.
105. Interview with Ariel Pablos-Mendez, May 2020.
106. Interview with Ariel Pablos-Mendez, May 2020.
107. A. Pablos-Mendez, M. C. Raviglione, "A new world health era", *Global Health: Science and Practice*, 2018, p. 3.
108. Interview with Richard Horton, August 2020.
109. Interview with Amina Muhammed, August 2021.
110. Interview with Suprotik Basu, July 2021.
111. Interview with Bob Orr, July 2021.
112. R. Lane, "Profile: Tore Godal: Quiet colossus of global health", *Lancet*, 14 December 2019, 394 (10215), p. 2142.
113. Interview with Monique Vledder, May 2021.
114. G. Brown, *Seven Ways to Change the World: How to Fix the Most Pressing Problems We Face* (London: Simon & Schuster, 2021), p. 222.

6 How Ebola Created the Coalition for Epidemic Preparedness Innovations (CEPI)

> . . . having coronavirus get going just as the Ebola outbreak is ending is like having Grendel's mother coming for Beowulf after he'd finally dispatched Grendel.[1]
>
> Sir Richard Peto[2]

The Ebola virus disease epidemic that broke out in West Africa in December 2013 entered a dramatic phase in the summer of 2014. Following 1711 reported cases and 932 recorded deaths, on 8 August, the WHO acknowledged that the outbreak was a public health emergency of international concern.[3] Major epidemics can be as politically destabilising as wars; they spread chaos, and the potential of the bat-borne virus to bring about a catastrophic loss of life led the UN Security Council to declare the Ebola epidemic a threat to international peace and security. As the deadly virus exposed the failings in the international community's ability to respond effectively, Tore Godal, and many others, grew concerned that if the virus mutated to become more easily transmissible, then Ebola could spread to the rest of Africa and become a global pandemic. At the time, there was no licenced vaccine against Ebola virus disease and no treatments.

The first (or 'index') case of the Ebola filovirus epidemic was a two-year-old child from a small village near the town of Guékédou in the Forest Region of Guinea who, after a short and devastating illness, died on 28 December 2013.[4] In subsequent months, the infectious disease spread rapidly and exponentially into neighbouring Liberia and Sierra Leone, two of the poorest countries in the world. Historically, since the discovery of the disease in 1976, Ebola outbreaks had involved relatively small case numbers, occurring in isolated rural areas with low population densities, making it possible to prevent the infection from spreading out of control through a combination of contact tracing and quarantine measures. What was different in 2014 was that the disease had migrated to the densely populated cities of the region. Clearly, the world was not prepared for such a decisive and unprecedented public health emergency. With a case fatality rate as high as 89%,[5] Godal believed that it was essential to develop an Ebola vaccine as quickly as possible, in order, 'to be prepared for the worst'.[6] This led

DOI: 10.4324/9781003363859-7

to the WHO, the Wellcome Trust, pharmaceutical companies and Godal acting on behalf of the Norwegian government, to enter a race to develop a vaccine that would contain the spread of Ebola virus disease epidemic.

The Anatomy of the Ebola Virus Epidemic

The eponymous Ebola virus first struck humans living in northern Zaire (later renamed the Democratic Republic of the Congo) in 1976 in villages along the Ebola River.[7] The disease can spread through exposure to contaminated blood of infected humans, and the notoriously deadly infection causes grievous symptoms the most conspicuous being severe diarrhoea, vomiting and haemorrhagic fever. A major source of transmission was the skin of people who had died of the disease; alas, a cultural tradition in many of the affected countries was that mourners touched the bodies of the dead as a mark of respect. Its high fatality rate, combined with the lack of knowledge about the disease's natural history, gave rise to a 'fear and fascination attached to Ebola infection', and even the 'possibility of terrorist groups using Ebola as a biological weapon'.[8]

In 1977, the biologists Jean and Peter Medawar described a virus as a piece of nucleic acid wrapped in bad news.[9] This description became an overwhelming truism for Liberia, Sierra Leona and Guinea – the three unfortunate countries most affected by the Ebola epidemic – and, as a later scientific inquiry acknowledged, these nations, because of debilitating civil wars and weakened health systems were, 'perhaps the least equipped to respond to an epidemic or to support clinical research during an epidemic'.[10] The unprecedented outbreak, in such a vulnerable region, alarmed many infectious disease researchers within the global health community. One of the physician-scientists who felt that the epidemic was being neglected and underestimated was Ripley Ballou, a leading member of GlaxoSmithKline's (GSK's) pioneering RTS,S malaria vaccine programme. Having begun working on a malaria vaccine while serving as a physician in the US Army in the 1980s, Ballou understood just how formidable this relatively new human pathogen could be to global public health.

> What was different in 2014 was that previous outbreaks had been exclusively in remote areas of Central Africa. However, in West Africa there was an extensive transportation network with major trucking routes all along the coast involving lots of cross border movement of very different populations; and because the disease is so transmissible I felt that this outbreak was going to have a very different epidemiology than we had previously seen with Ebola.[11]

Serendipitously, Ballou was aware that GSK had earlier acquired the Italian biotechnology company Okairos, which had successfully developed a vaccine technology that used deactivated chimpanzee-derived adenoviruses that produced a very strong response against target diseases and for which they had very impressive protection data.[12] Sensing that GSK might be able to develop a novel Ebola vaccine using this new technology, Ballou sought to persuade his bosses to fully mobilise GSK's worldwide research network and set in motion a global response to what he believed could become a global catastrophe. However, at the beginning of 2014, the pharmaceutical industry's decision-making capacity was dependent upon international conventions.

> And they said, 'Oh that is very interesting, but we really can't do anything unless the WHO requests it, and without that, there is no way we are going to get this work prioritised'. That is when I called Marie-Paule Kieny at the WHO in Geneva.[13]

For almost a decade at the beginning of new millennium, Marie-Paule Kieny was the Director of the WHO Initiative for Vaccine Research. The disease portfolio of the Initiative included tropical diseases, HIV/AIDS, tuberculosis, malaria, meningitis, respiratory diseases, Japanese encephalitis, cervical cancer and measles.[14] Additionally, during the 2009–2010 H1N1 influenza pandemic, Kieny oversaw the WHO's pandemic vaccine deployment initiative, which lead the way for the delivery of 77 million doses of vaccine to 78 low- and middle-income countries to enable immunisation of health workers and priority populations. Moreover, because of Kieny's long-term association with the biotech industry, and research experience within the field of vaccinology, she knew Ripley Ballou well and respected his science and insightful understanding of the threats to global public health. 'It must have been around March in 2014, when Ripley Ballou contacted me', Kieny recounted later, 'and he said that GSK had acquired a candidate Ebola vaccine, and asked if the WHO was interested?' At the time, Kieny was Assistant Director-General for Health Systems and was no longer working in the area of infectious diseases. However, when she spoke with her infectious disease colleagues, they seemed somewhat dismissive of Ballou's offer and confident that there was no impending danger. 'They told me to, "just go away, this will be gotten rid of through conventional measures". As it was not my area of work, I said "Okay". Later, I got back to Rip with the answer. "No, no interest"'.[15]

First gradually, and then suddenly, the crisis exposed the weaknesses in the WHO's leadership and capabilities. Despite the clear evidence that the outbreak was decimating communities and overwhelming local health systems,[16] the WHO failed to mobilise personnel, materials and finance with sufficient speed and urgency. This administrative paralysis, together with a lack of local leadership served to exacerbate the crisis and, as the pandemic entered the dramatic months of the summer, Marie-Paul Kieny saw an opportunity to take control and build a partnership to deliver humanitarian assistance, and develop and test experimental vaccines within the lifetime of the epidemic.

At the beginning of August, many people in the WHO and in other organisations were on vacation, so I replaced a number of colleagues and that is how I became involved. It immediately became clear that this epidemic was going in the wrong direction, and the first thing that I did was to set up a meeting with ethicists to discuss whether it was acceptable to use untested medicine in populations in the context of the epidemic.[17]

Following Kieny's accession to power and responsibility, the Director-General of the WHO, Margaret Chan, then chose her to lead the WHO campaign to develop drugs and vaccines against Ebola.

Two thousand kilometres north of the WHO's Geneva headquarters, Tore Godal paced the floor of his office in Oslo. He was so concerned about the inadequacies of the world's response that he had telephoned Peter Smith, a long-time collaborator from the early days of vaccine development at TDR. As one of the world's leading tropical disease epidemiologists and vaccine trialists, Smith served on a number of international committees and was a Governor of the Wellcome Trust. Therefore, Godal believed that if anyone could identify the most promising vaccine candidates against Ebola, it would be his global public health colleague. Throughout the month of August, high-level political meetings had been taking place at the WHO with representatives from the affected countries, the United States, United Kingdom and France, and both the National Institutes of Health (NIH) and the Centers for Disease Control and Prevention (CDC) presented plans to evaluate the efficacy of Ebola vaccines in West Africa.[18] By the end of August, the WHO had decided that in such exceptional circumstances it would be ethical to evaluate unregistered therapeutic interventions in people with the Ebola virus disease.[19] Following this crucial announcement, in early September, Peter Smith attended a WHO meeting to assess Ebola vaccine development and he was able to describe to Godal the scientific characteristics of three vaccine candidates. The first was a recombinant viral-vectored vaccine based on vesicular stomatitis virus (VSV) coated with Ebola surface protein. VSV is replication competent, meaning that it can spread throughout the body after vaccination but does not cause disease. The other vaccines were DNA based and were replication-deficient recombinant simian adenoviral-vectored. Being replication-deficient means that it cannot spread to other cells and so will not cause an ongoing infection. From the vantage point, a tropical disease immunologist, Godal immediately saw the advantages of the VSV-ZEBOV vaccine (Merck NewLink Genetics), even though it necessitated a complex cold-chain deployment system to keep it at the requisite low temperature. Unlike the Chimpanzee adenovirus vaccine ChAd3 EBOZ (GlaxoSmithKleine), it did not require *two* injections, which would be a difficult undertaking during an outbreak. Both the vaccines had shown the ability to project macaques against the Ebola virus but neither had undergone human trials. With each passing week, as infections levels and death rates increased so too did Godal's determination to strengthen the WHO's efforts to control the epidemic; to achieve this objective, he knew that the most reliable way to identify the efficacy – or dangers – of drugs, vaccines and other investigational products[20] was to carry out randomised controlled trials. The science of statistics forms a crucial part of decision-making in the modern world, and over the autumn of 2014 Godal mobilised Norwegian development aid funding and scientific expertise to augment the life and death choices that affected countries, pharmaceutical companies and the WHO were to make.

The Ring Vaccination Clinical Trial

Under the dynamic leadership of Marie-Paule Kieny, coordination and cooperation became the new leitmotifs of the WHO's campaign to end the epidemic in West Africa. As a result, the Ebola vaccine trials were designed, approved and implemented at a speed that belied the disorganisation in the WHO's delayed response to the crisis.[21] The planning and conducting of clinical studies during an epidemic raised important and understandable ethical considerations. Some doubted whether it was even ethical to conduct clinical trials in the midst of a public health emergency. Meanwhile, others, including members of the WHO Ethics Working Group, argued that there was an ethical obligation to conduct research during the epidemic.[22] Throughout September – as the epidemic reached its peak – the ethics of trial design was hotly debated.[23,24] On 29 September, Kieny invited Godal to a meeting she had convened in Geneva to coordinate the planned clinical trials for candidate Ebola vaccines. The dilemma centred on the question of what was the best trial design to test efficacy. All of the assembled experts knew that it would be a hugely demanding exercise to carry out clinical trials under such difficult conditions, but ultimately it was the most reliable method to evaluate whether the Ebola vaccines were effective against the virus. Before enrolling participants in human trials, a vaccine will have undergone extensive tests in the laboratory, but ultimately only a trial in the patient can give the answer to its efficacy or warn of its dangers.[25] Trials to test vaccine efficacy are called phase III trials; typically, these trials are blinded randomised placebo-controlled trials – this means that half the people being vaccinated receive the vaccine, and half receive a placebo inoculation (i.e. an inert substance, such as a saline injection). However, because Ebola has such a high mortality rate, it was argued by some researchers that it was unethical to conduct a randomised controlled trial (RCT) in which people had a 50% chance of being given a hypothetically protective vaccine or a 50% of being denied immunogenic protection. The ensuing discussions Kieny remembers as being 'quite tense'[26] and determining the choice of the control arm proved to one of the most contentious points in designing Ebola vaccine trials.[27] The founder of statistical inference, RA Fisher, once famously wrote this damning review of a study that lacked sufficient scientific rigour: 'That is not an experiment you have there, that's an experience'.[28] Thus, all of the researchers wanted to ensure that the methodology used in their respective clinical trials would provide reliable and verifiable findings. There-fore, to get the right answer in an epidemiological study, researchers need to take great care in the planning, execution and publication of the experiment. One pragmatic alternative for a phase III trial is a step-wedge design, which takes into account that the disease outbreak is widespread and the intervention is given to participants over a designated timescale, either as individuals or in clusters. As all of the participants would ultimately receive the Ebola vaccine, the design appealed to those who 'opposed placebos or active controls for ethical reasons'.[29]

In October, a meeting was held at a critical stage in the WHO's efforts to accel-erate the development of candidate Ebola vaccines which could immediately enter clinical evaluation. Following passionate deliberations between health spe-cialists and regulators, the NIH opted to test for safety and efficacy in a traditional placebo-controlled RCT in Liberia, while the CDC elected to deploy a two-arm immediate and delayed vaccination approach (stepped wedge design) with indi-vidual randomisation in Sierra Leone. The WHO welcomed these north–south partnerships; nonetheless, it became increasingly clear to Marie-Paule Kieny,

> that no research agency was interested in doing a clinical trial in Guinea. And of course, Guinea found that unacceptable. They were the biggest country and the first country affected and they thought that they should be a part of the solution.[30]

This disturbing omission served as a powerful rallying call to Godal, and Kieny, to build a partnership, 'in protest against the Americans',[31] that would fill the experimental void.[32] After a flurry of coordination and communication side meetings, alliances were quickly formed between leading medical academ-ics including Peter Smith and Mike Levine, together with representatives from the WHO, Médecins Sans Frontières (MSF), Merck, GSK and the Norwegian Institute of Public Health. Godal's influence was decisive in the early days of the working group's formation. 'We felt something had to be done', the urgency of the crisis still discernible in Godal's voice some seven years later,

> and Marie-Paule was keen to get a trial going in Guinea. I was attracted to the idea, even though it would be a gamble, because the weak infrastructure of the country would make it a challenge to carry out, but on the other hand, I thought Guinea would be the country where the epidemic would last longest. In October I told Marie-Paule that we would like to invest in a vaccine trial.[33]

Behind the scenes, using customary subtlety, Godal was able to channel the close historical and emotional ties that Norway had to the WHO, and global immunisation campaigns, to secure US$2.5 million from GLOBVAC, a fund he had asked Prime Minister Jens Stoltenberg to set up in 2006, to support Nor-wegian led research on vaccine development and deployment. This funding, however, came with one condition; it would require a Norwegian investigator to lead the project. The prerequisite of securing the assistance of an experienced practitioner in international randomised controlled trials led Godal to the eminent epidemiologist Halvor Sommerfelt at the University of Bergen. Coincidentally, Sommerfelt's group had recently attained the prestigious *Centres of Excellence* status, together with a substantial increase in un-earmarked finance, from the Norwegian Research Council. Timing is as determining a factor in global health as it is in other aspects of human endeavour, and on this occasion, Sommerfelt declined the offer to lead the vaccine trial in Guinea, as he felt an understandable obligation to concentrate his efforts on developing the *Centres of Excellence* programme. Nevertheless, and acting in a spirit of solidarity, Halvor Sommerfelt suggested to Godal that he contact the distinguished infectious diseases physician John-Arne Røttingen, at the Public Health Institute, as John-Arne had control of abundant human and financial resources that could feed into the Ebola trial. It turned out to be a good choice. Although John-Arne Røttingen was not a trialist, and indeed had never run a RCT, he had a lot of international experience, including working with the WHO. He also had one overriding quality, the ability to get things done even under the most challenging circumstances. John-Arne Røttingen said yes.

Even with the recruitment of John-Arne Røttingen, funding was still an issue. With the onset of autumn, Godal's ability to raise additional monies became somewhat easier, according to a study by Antonie de Bengy Puyvallée, when the Norwegian government began to evaluate Ebola as a major biosecurity threat, particularly after the repatriation of a 'health worker infected with Ebola' to Oslo in October 2014.[34] Within days, Godal was able to secure a further US$1 million from the Ministry of Foreign Affairs, and this catalysed several other donors, the most important being the Wellcome Trust, which via a series of multi-million pound grants hastened the plans to combat the outbreak. The Trust's Director, Jeremy Farrar, wanted to speed up epidemic emergency response and for the 'trials to happen quickly, and in an ethically and scientifically robust setting, to find out if any new Ebola treatments actually work'.[35] Just as valuable as the purchasing power of Norway that Godal was instrumental in bringing to the trial, he also brought what Marie-Paule Kieny describes as, 'a lot of added credibility to the project when he gave his support and backing'.[36] These commitments enabled the WHO Consortium (VEBCON) to conduct phase I or first-in-human trials of the rVSV-ZEBOV vaccine simultaneously in Switzerland, Germany, Kenya and Gabon. One remarkable feature of the rVSV-ZEBOV vaccine is that its existence and preparedness for clinical trials was fortuitous, as it was not originally developed for humanitarian purposes, or as part of a public health response for populations in areas vulnerable to the natural emergence of the disease, but rather, 'to assist in countering potential future bioterrorist attacks'.[37] Scientists at the Public Health Agency of Canada initially developed the vaccine candidate in 2000 with additional funding coming from the Canadian Safety and Security Program and the Department of Defence – and, coincidentally, Ebola happened to be on the list of pathogens that the military thought had the potential for bioterrorism use one day. In 2010, NewLink Genetics Corporation, a small biotechnology company based in Ames, Iowa acquired the commercial rights to the rVSV-EBOV, and in November 2014, Merck & Co., Inc., licenced the vaccine and assumed the responsibility for efforts to research, develop, manufacture and distribute the vaccine. The perpetual struggle between people and pathogens was about to enter a dramatic new phase.

Because of the urgency of the Ebola outbreak, the combined forces of private-sector innovation and public-sector political leadership melded to build a nexus of trust, and forge partnerships so prodigious that the clinical development of the vaccine proceeded in record time, taking less than a year to achieve what under normal circumstance would take a decade. By December, the Guinea vaccine Consortium, comprising academics, physicians, scientists, epidemiologists and experts from Merck, the WHO, Norway, Canada, Guinea and Doctors without Borders, were ready to turn their attentions to the design of the clinical trial. The French epidemiology group Doctors without Borders (MSF Médecins Sans Frontières) who had previously deployed the meningitis and cholera vaccines in Guinea and brought that crucial practical field experience to the group argued that it would not be possible to carry out a trial randomised at the individual level. At this point, Peter Smith proposed a cluster randomised trial, and when the ethical aspect of the non-vaccinated group came up, Godal suggested, 'that vaccination could follow after a defined period'.[38] As Marie-Paule Kieny recalled, 'this was group work, with people standing in front of a white board saying, "what do you think of that?" Eventually we came up with the idea of a ring vaccination trial'.[39] Ring vaccination was a pragmatic approach that adapted the extremely successful strategy pioneered by Bill Foege during the global smallpox eradication campaign in the 1970s. With their methodology, they isolated smallpox patients by vaccinating family members and other close contacts, creating a concentric ring barrier around the disease. In Guinea, the Ring Vaccination method works by identifying Ebola virus disease cases, then rapidly immunising all of their close contacts, as well as the contacts of those contacts. That group of people forms a *ring* around the initial case. The phase III Ring Vaccination trial,[40] *Ebola ça suffit* (Ebola, this is enough!) began on 23 March 2015 and was conducted by the WHO, Médecins Sans Frontières and the Norwegian Institute of Public Health. In the clinical trial, approximately 5,800 participants, who met the protocol inclusion criteria and the definition of a 'contact' or 'contact of a contact' of a laboratory-confirmed Ebola virus disease, were vaccinated with an intramuscular injection of rVSV-ZEBOZ following randomisation to either immediate or delayed (21 days) vaccination arms.[41] This replaced the classical placebo regime, but the trial was still a randomised controlled trial. 'We knew it was a race against time', remembered John-Arne Røttingen, who was the chair of the trial's steering group, 'and that the trial had to be implemented under the most challenging circumstances'.[42] The three leaders of the trial, John-Arne Røttingen, Maria-Paule Kieny and Ana-Maria Henao-Restrepo, oversaw the trial on the ground in Guinea.[43] For too long, health workers had been unprotected against the Ebola pathogen, but now with the prospect of deploying a vaccine that could protect lives and break chains of transmission, the Médecins Sans Frontières vaccination teams worked tirelessly. These frontline workers were undeterred by the considerable operational challenges that they faced in the field, including community resistance, difficulty reaching remote hamlets, having to transport the vaccine at very low temperatures and, not to be forgotten, undertaking a clinical trial during a deadly epidemic. These were the truly indispensable people in the Ring Vaccination trial. They travelled to inaccessible villages, where they erected treatment tents in the stultifying summer heat, while simultaneously explaining everything about the vaccine and its administration, building trust and administering the precious vaccine that they had kept refrigerated in RTIC coolers. Then, late in the evening, the vaccinators would repack the treatment tents and leave the village for a long gruelling drive back to their base. This schedule was systematically repeated for each ring in the trial; that they were able to maintain that with such scientific precision, against a lethal infection, stands as a testament to their resolution.

Godal's belief that the Ebola outbreak would last longest in Guinea proved correct, and the Ring Vaccination trial, because of its swift and thorough implementation managed in the marvellously evocative phrase of Marie-Paule Kieny, 'to catch the tail of the epidemic'.[44] Indeed, to the expert eye, the trial's design provided early and convincing evidence of the vaccine's efficacy. One of the experts examining the evolving evidence was the epidemiologist Swati Gupta, an integral member of the Merck's Ebola vaccine team: 'Even before the efficacy data came out, we knew that after the ring vaccination was occurring in different villages, you could see the disease go away'.[45] It very soon became apparent that the vaccine gave protection against the Ebola virus within 10 days of administering for both the intervention and the control groups. By the end of June, three months after the trial had begun, the oversight group, which included among its members the world-renowned epidemiologist and clinical trialist, Richard Peto, informed the investigators that the study had reached a significant finding. By the summer of 2015, the intensive efforts to bring the virus under control using contact tracing, quarantine and hygiene measures were paying dividends, and case numbers were low and falling.[46] This reality, together with the high-quality efficacy data, led the Ring Vaccination trial's Data and Safety Monitoring Board (DSMB) to recommend ending randomisation and that all subsequent contacts received immediate vaccination.[47]

Trial Results

The results of the phase III *Ebola ça Suffit* trial were published (online) on 31 July 2015, in *The Lancet* and generated, remarkable interim findings,[48] indicating that the rVSV-ZEBOV vaccine is highly efficacious (100%, 95% confidence interval: 75–100). The audacity of the international community's ability to launch such a novel clinical trial, and the determination of the Guinean people to conduct the experiment in the midst of one of the worst public health crises in decades, prompted an admiring editorial in *The Lancet*.

> That such a trial was even possible is a testament not only to the skill of the research teams but also to the commitment of communities to defeating an epidemic that has devastated their nation. Over 90 percent of the study's staff was from Guinea. Before this work, no clinical trial on this scale had ever been performed in the country.

One prestigious US review even went as far as using a sporting metaphor to represent the trial's achievement to its readership. 'Among all of the therapeutic and vaccine trials conducted in West Africa during the outbreak, the ring vaccination trial came the closest to fulfilling the hope for a clinical trial "home run" (or a "six," its cricket equivalent)'.[49] Indeed, the *Ebola ça Suffit* trial was the *only* vaccine trial completed during the outbreak. These laudatory comments describing the vaccine as a global public good should, to continue the sporting allegory, have been sufficient to knock any criticisms, 'out of the park'. However, as the nineteenth-century philosopher Friedrich Nietzsche famously declared, 'there are no facts, only interpretations'.[50] When the results were published, Marie-Paule Kieny thought that

> everyone would be happy, but it was terrible, we were pilloried. People said, 'this is not a trial, this is a study'. But, we were lucky because Ana Maria Henao-Restrepo, the leader of the trial, was very experienced in clinical research, and had previously been involved in vaccine deployment in Africa. And, of course, Richard Peto, who played an important role in the statistical analysis, brought the trial credibility.[51]

Some of the criticism focused on the cluster randomised design being less efficient than an individually randomised design,[52] while others raised ethical and interpretational concerns.[53-54] To the dispassionate observer, the reality was that the ring vaccination trial was a miraculous undertaking; in less than one year, the vaccine had been successfully developed, distributed and tested during a devastating epidemic. Throughout the tumultuous months of the epidemic when the Guinea vaccine Consortium was forming, Godal was constantly available to support Marie-Paule Kieny in her role at the WHO.

More than anything, Tore is a doer. He has the power to move things forward, and he would not let doubt contaminate our minds. The other essential person was Jeremy Farrar; he had the capacity to get money out of the Wellcome Trust, which was instrumental in allowing the clinical trial to happen. Tore and Jeremy were really the godfathers of the project.[55]

Crucially, the trial was peer reviewed by six referees, working at two study stations, over 2 weeks; their impartial analysis of the measurable impacts on people's lives meant that, 'the trial', became in the judgement of John-Arne Røttingen, 'a huge success'.[56]

Another medical scientist who played a decisive role in the development of the vaccine was Mark Feinberg, a chief public health science officer at Merck. In this role, he helped to upscale the production of the vaccine from the original vials delivered to the WHO and presented the synchronised data to the regulators in a convincing way that allowed the US Food and Drug Administration (FDA) and the European Medicines Agency (EMA) to licence the vaccine and give it 'emergency authorisation'. Thus, according to the physician-scientist, Mark Feinberg,

the trial in Guinea validated a critical tool for our ability to respond to Ebola outbreaks. It grew out of our initial discussions where Tore, as the champion of both public health and equity considerations, was what ultimately generated the efficacy data for the Ebola vaccine. If that study had not happened, our understanding of vaccines, our ability to deploy an efficacious vaccine, and our knowledge of how to undertake a ring vaccination strategy, which is a key element now, would not have happened.[57]

The ring vaccination trial, which deciphered many mysteries, had a complex historical evolution and if it had not been for one decisive factor, Swati Gupta thinks that things could have very much worse than they were.

What people don't know is that at the time the outbreak happened there were already GMP (good manufacturing practice) clinical doses of the vaccine in the freezer otherwise we couldn't have gone straight into trial at that time. If it had been another type of Ebola (there are 5 types) we would have been in big trouble.

Is it human nature that as a species we don't necessarily prepare for things, and that it is more usual to respond after the fact? Against a lethal infection, a lack of preparedness could prove catastrophic.

Acknowledging this reality brings us back to the dilemma facing Ripley Ballou and his GSK colleagues in the early months of 2014. Fearing that the epidemic in

West Africa was 'getting out of hand', their willingness to fast-track safety and immunogenicity clinical phase I studies was dependent upon the WHO declaring a public health emergency of international concern. 'Once that happened in August, and the WHO pulled the trigger', reflected a thoughtful Ripley Ballou, 'we were able to put together a crash team at GSK to work with the NIH, and with Adrian Hill's team at Oxford University to accelerate progress on our Ebola vaccine ChAd3'.[58] One member of the Oxford team was the vaccinologist, Sarah Gilbert, and in a recent publication she vividly describes, 'what went right, and then what went wrong, in our response to the Ebola outbreak'.[59] In September 2014, the GSK ChAd3 vaccine and the rVSV vaccine were the only candidates that met the WHO criteria; and the aim and expectation had been that the two vaccines would be tested for efficacy at the same time in different locations. However, with the rVSV vaccine bringing the outbreak under control, the ChAd3 vaccine was never tested for efficacy. Sarah Gilbert saw the problem as a 'lack of preparation' and 'while the discussions about the design of the efficacy study were going on, around 5,000 people became infected and more than 2,000 died'. Gilbert is eloquent in her defence of those hard-working health care workers, trialists and lab-based researchers who labour tirelessly in the most challenging of circumstances; she sees the problem as a lack of preparation. 'In truth, despite having known about Ebola virus since 1976, and despite having invested in vaccine development over many years, the world was not ready in 2014 to test a vaccine against Ebola. The response was simply not adequate'.[60] The 2013–2016 Ebola epidemic resulted in over 28,600 cases and more than 11,300 deaths, cost an estimated \$59 billion, and revealed significant shortcomings in the functions and performance of the international public health system.[61] The world's inadequate response to Ebola was a wake-up call and a turning point for GlaxoSmithKline and for Ripley Ballou after his experience of working through the scientific emergency.

> The reason our vaccine did not go forward was we could not scale-up manufacturing in the timeframe that we had. We could not provide the 300,000 doses necessary. Ebola had a very disruptive impact on GSK; we put in hundreds of millions of dollars in expenses and personnel time. Remember GSK had responded to the influenza epidemic in 2009, pulled out of the stops, made vast numbers of vaccine doses available, and interrupted other programmes, and we did the same with Ebola. At that point, we at GSK said, *'We can't do this again. There needs to be a better way of doing this'.*[62]

A Global Problem Requires a Global Response

The Ebola epidemic was a potent viral warning that infectious diseases represent a deadly threat to global public health in terms of lives lost and in causing catastrophic economic disruption. To Godal the epidemic served as a wake-up call that highlighted the need for the world to be better prepared for future crises, and that the WHO's operational model for outbreak vigilance and response was demonstrably obsolete. As early as the summer of 2015, he saw that it was essential to transform the global health landscape and he launched his campaign for change at the World Health Assembly in Geneva at the end of May. The World Health Assembly is the governing body of the WHO and is positioned at the intersection of medical science and politics where policies and programmes evolve, and where intellectual skirmishes can often occur. 'Tore challenged me at the World Health Assembly', Marie-Paule Kieny recalls, 'he said, "You, the WHO, have to put a plan together". So, he challenged me and after this we started to work on what is called the WHO Blueprint on Epidemic Preparedness'.[63] The R&D Blueprint would bring together scientists, public health specialists and regulators in an emergency fast-track research into diagnostics, treatments and vaccines.

At the beginning of the century, Godal had shown that the secret of GAVI's success was its unique public–private business model and its focus on innovation and scale, while expressly seeking to protect people against both endemic diseases and those with epidemic potential. However, there are no vaccines against many infectious diseases, and no market incentive for manufacturers to develop them. To remedy this deficiency, during the summer of 2015, Godal strategically deployed his political and scientific influence to fill the critical gap that existed and ensure that the world would have the vaccines it needs.[64] His was not a lone voice, and support for a global research and financing mechanism was growing, with calls for a $2 billion fund for vaccine development for pandemics.[65] In July 2015, Jeremy Farrar, together with Adel Mahmoud, a former president of vaccines at Merck & Co., and Stanley Plotkin, the celebrated vaccinologist, proposed the development of an international fund to carry vaccines from their conception in academic or government laboratories to development and licensure by industry.[66] As the authors emphasised, this translational journey was so precarious that few vaccine candidates safely navigated a way through the so-called valley of death the critical stages from the laboratory bench to a phase I clinical trial, and proof of concept in terms of protective immune responses. Their article ended with a warning from history regarding the dangers of neglecting tropical diseases that had pandemic potential.

> The lesson we take from the Ebola crisis is that disease prevention should not be held back by lack of money at a critical juncture when a relatively modest, strategic investment could save thousands of lives and billions of dollars further down the line.[67]

In his efforts to ensure that the world would be better prepared for future outbreaks, Jeremy Farrar contacted Godal, because he knew that if he was to succeed in raising the US$2 billion needed to develop vaccines against epidemic outbreaks, it would need to be a global effort, requiring trusted and effective part-nerships. This phone call from Farrar to Godal forms a decisive moment in the history of global public health. For his part, Godal thought that $2 billion 'was very ambitious' but he understood the paramount need for an entity to develop vaccines much faster against epidemic outbreaks. 'Jeremy's call galvanised in me', Godal recalled, 'a belief that we could mobilise a sufficiently broad-based support for action'.[68]

On 14 August, in a perceptive and challenging article in *Science*, Klenk and Becker wrote that 'many lives might have been saved if the phase I clinical studies in which the safety and immunogenicity of the vaccines against Ebola virus was assessed' had been completed earlier.[69] The need to speed up epidemic emergency response motivated John-Arne Røttingen and Godal to write a rejoin-der letter in *Science* in which they listed four elements that could have enabled earlier implementation and conclusion of their ring vaccination trial. In closing, they signposted a historic, global, way forward.

> This means that in future, analogous situations, an international blueprint for R&D preparedness and response could reduce the total time of implementing and concluding phase 3 vaccine trials during an outbreak. . . . We hope the world will support such a framework for better international coordination of R&D for epidemic emergencies.

Among the lessons learned by Godal and Røttingen from the Ebola outbreak was the need to have vaccines available against other viruses at the onset of an epidemic.

In early September, Godal met with the Norwegian Foreign Minister, Børge Brende to discuss strategies to improve health and education policies relating to the Sustainable Development Goals (SDGs). The meeting was to prove a happy conjuncture, as the Foreign Minister was as equally committed to establishing a new entity to develop vaccines against neglected infectious diseases as he was to his government's policy of Worldwide Education for Girls.

> When I told Børge Brende that we needed to fund a new initiative to develop new vaccines and deliver them at speed, to everyone who needs them, he was immediately fired up and said that he would commit 200 million NOK per year to the project.[70]

Børge Brende was an ardent supporter of global public health, gaining a visceral understanding of the damage caused by the Ebola epidemic when he travelled to Liberia in 2014, together with Rajiv Shah of USAID. They visited the capital city, Monrovia, where the healthcare system had been completely overwhelmed, and people suffering from the disease were being stigmatised. 'A lot of myths about the disease were swirling around', Børge Brende recalled with echoing clarity,

> and it was the most importing undertaking. I will never forget when President Ellen Johnson Sirleaf, hugged Raj and myself and said, 'so glad to see you giving support and solidarity'. To see the amount of despair that Ebola could create was something unforgettable.[71]

Operating in a liminal, transformative space, between '*realpolitik*'[72] and science, when Godal left Børge Brende's office, he decided that he would keep the figure of 200 million a secret, as he knew that it was essential when negotiating with other donors to know precisely what level of contribution the Norwegian government could match. This was important, as the concept of 'matching grants' is attractive to potential donors as it contributes to a belief that *their* money will get them that extra mile. Godal's forte is that he understands the art of influence and persuasion, and as his former Norad colleague Helga Fogstad believes this lies 'in an understanding of who the players are, and how to get them around a table, and how to play your cards in order to get the game going'.[73] As Godal walked out of the Ministry of Foreign Affairs, he was comforted in the knowledge that he had mobilised the first government commitment to fund a new vaccine development initiative. He, however, was less sanguine about navigating the way ahead, knowing that for the initiative to succeed, it would require all of his immanent spirit, political astuteness and every molecule of his legendary resilience.

The Development of the Coalition for Epidemic Preparedness Innovations (CEPI)

Any attempt to establish what was in effect a multilateral start-up was inevitably going to be criticised for lacking legitimacy. Fortunately, for Godal and the other promotors of change, the Ebola catastrophe had caused, in the striking phrase of Peter Piot, a co-discoverer of the Ebola virus in 1976, 'an epidemic of reports'.[74] One of the earliest and most powerful of these condemnatory reports was, 'Will Ebola change the game? Ten essential reforms before the next pandemic. The report of the Harvard-LSHTM Independent Panel on the Response to Ebola'.[75] Led by Surie Moon and Peter Piot, the report emphasised how Ebola had exposed weaknesses and shortcoming in the functions and performance of the international global health system, while at the same time taking a figurative sledgehammer to the WHO's status as the institutional pillar for global health security. 'The reputation and credibility of WHO has suffered a particularly fierce blow'.[76] The Panel set out a detailed manifesto of how to reinforce the fragile global system of outbreak response, and among the essential reforms called for was to 'establish a global facility to finance, accelerate, and prioritise research and development' for the vaccines that are crucial to health security, when commercial incentives are inappropriate.[77] The Panel was chaired by Peter Piot, the then Director of the London School of Hygiene and Tropical Medicine:

> the advantage of that report is that it was a global type committee, with members of the Panel from Africa, whereas most of the other committees were more donor-driven. And the Ebola outbreak in West Africa was a wake-up call and the beginning of interest in pandemic preparedness.[78]

Throughout the final months of 2015, the multiplier effect of WHO's credibility being 'battered',[79] together with orchestrated calls for a new organisation to develop vaccines for public health purposes, shaped a decisive moment, which enabled Godal, and like-minded colleagues to bring together a collection of eclectic groups determined to improve the global health architecture of epidemic and pandemic response.

As one of the great survivors in global public health, Godal's longevity is due in part to his very concrete, transactional outlook. Before starting a new initiative, he needed to be sure there was a problem to address, pinpoint a concrete action of what to do and then do it. As a systems thinker and a builder, Godal sought to construct overlapping circles of interests and expertise that would change the structure of global health to remedy the threat of potential pandemics. His challenge would be to try to keep multiple stakeholders happy that align on the objective but might not necessarily agree on the mechanisms of achieving their collective ambition. Once Godal informed Jeremy Farrar at the Wellcome Trust that the Norwegian government was interested in the project, they then started to think about the shape and form of the organisation, together with the identity of other groups that could give added legitimacy to their nascent project. A critical step in the transformation of global health was the talks held in Oslo, in October 2015, which became the WHO R&D Blueprint for Action to Prevent Epidemics.[80] At this gathering, the participants agreed to eschew any distractive R&D involvement in diagnostics and therapeutics and instead focus solely on vaccines with limited market prospects. Meanwhile, a subtle recalibration in global health governance took place when individuals from the Wellcome Trust, World Economic Forum, the Gates Foundation, the Norwegian Institute of Public Health and the Norwegian Ministry of Foreign Affairs, were selected to form a Core Group to take the concept forward. Marie-Paule Kieny, WHO Assistant Director-General for Health Systems and Innovation, sees the Oslo assemblage as integral to the development of the new organisation. 'CEPI is the brainchild of the Blueprint. The idea of CEPI came in that pre-blueprint meeting. It wasn't called CEPI at the time, but it came at that moment in Oslo'.[81] Moreover, Kiney's involvement is a testament the close interconnectedness of the individuals and groups who worked on the Ebola outbreak and those shaping the design and philosophy of the new initiative. It showed how one global health challenge is not merely about that specific challenge but is integral to the intellectual and practical bedrock of another. Kiney, who ran the ring vaccination trial for the WHO, later became an 'observer' member of the CEPI Interim Board. John-Arne Røttingen led the steering group of the ring vaccination trial in Guinea and would later head the CEPI Secretariat during the first phase[82] of its development. In addition, Mark Feinberg, who helped expedite the development of the Ebola vaccine, was recruited to Merck by Adel Mahmoud and would later act as chair of the Scientific Advisory Board that selected the choice of vaccine platforms for CEPI to pursue. At the apex of the structure was Jeremy Farrar and Godal, both of whom were involved in the West Africa trials, the genesis of the WHO Blueprint and the co-equal progenitors of the CEPI ideal. As clinicians with vast field research experience, they shared a similar perspective on the needs of global public health in the twenty-first century. They believed that 'the world needed science'[83] and for academia and industry to find a mechanism that would enabled them to work effectively together against known and unknown pathogens while retaining a 'strong thread of social justice'.[84]

One long-standing colleague in infectious disease research who Godal was eager to amalgamate into their plans was Peter Piot, who had represented the UN Secretary-General for the establishment of the Global Fund to Fight AIDS/ tuberculosis and malaria. Godal knew that while on the one hand the collection of stakeholders had much in common, inevitably, there was 'turf to be protected' and his experiences as the first CEO of GAVI served as a warning against complacency. At the beginning of November 2015, the first physical meeting of the still nameless organisation took place in Dublin, Ireland, with the formidable figure of Peter Piot chairing proceedings. 'In the beginning', Piot recalls from his home in Belgium,

> people said, 'this is impossible!' Tore was one of the only people who believed firmly in it. Because of my work on AIDS, I was convinced that we could only find a solution when all of those who are part of the solution are under the same roof, all in the tent together.[85]

As Jeremy Farrar looked around the cavernous room at the occasionally recalcitrant, but in the main supportive assembled representatives of the pharmaceutical industry, academia, think tanks and philanthropy he grew increasingly convinced of a phenomenon that he recognised had the capacity to alter the planning and organisation of biomedical science.

> I think that like most things in life and it certainly is in global health, that there are these *moments* when certain things happen, and constellations of the right eclectic groups come together that turn something into a decisive moment in the life of an idea or an institution.[86]

Even so, keeping these multiple stakeholders happy took an immense investment in understanding the psychology of why people and countries make certain decisions. Keeping those who were in the tent happy took persuasion, and the art of persuasion was Godal's forte. He practised this quiet art by being humble, persistent and persuasive; he also instinctively knew how to manoeuvre in the unforgiving non-evidence-based world of politics. In fact, Godal had become so adept at reasoned persuasion that in the opinion of Jeremy Farrar, he had perfected it into an art form.

> Tore is a survivor, and he understands the dark arts of influence probably better than anyone else, and he has been lucky, but you make your own luck. He has been in a country that is really committed to the global public good. Norway stands out as being extraordinary, but that doesn't happen by chance, it has been because of people like Tore.[87]

During the final weeks of 2015, many of these collective aberrant moments had created a powerful impetus to redesign the world's response to, and preparation for, the next pandemic. This was the key selling point for establishing CEPI. By demonstrating that GSK and Merck had developed Ebola vaccines in peacetime, Godal and others wanted to show that it was therefore possible to be ready and prepared ahead of an outbreak that might threaten global public health and security. Of course, the problem for the vaccine companies, governed as they are by commercial imperatives, was how could they take the risk of preparing for an outbreak with all the incumbent research costs involved, while there was no guarantee that an expensively prepared vaccine was even going to be used or required. John-Arne Røttingen viewed this dilemma as essentially, 'an insurance problem', and it became clear to many that what was required was an organisation that could pool resources and make decisions. The discussions of how to frame CEPI took place during the formative days of October and November with various theoretical ideas whirling around the room, creating action and reaction, position and opposition, into the maelstrom John-Arne Røttingen advocated his own conceptual outlook for the future.

> The debate was should we design CEPI as a global health development or position it as a security measure? I was of the opinion that it should be a global health security issue, and I framed it as an insurance mechanism, that countries needed to pay their premiums and be a part of this.[88]

All of the time, Godal continued to build his circles of connectivity linking the worlds of finance, science and politics. This led to the World Economic Forum taking an interest in the evolving plans, and their offer to use the convening power of their annual meeting in Davos, in January 2016, to bring all the interested stakeholders together to formulate a strategy for the emerging organisation.

Godal understood that in the global health context, often with a long-standing problem, elements of the solution already exist, and what he was particularly good at was bringing those people and their institutions to collaborate to solve problems. Sometimes, it was about leveraging existing institutions as with the Global Financing Facility at the World Bank, and on other occasions, it required creating a new institution as with GAVI. The setting for initiating the yearlong strategic plan to create this new institution was Davos, global capitalisms spiritual home, positioned high in the Swiss Alps. At the World Economic Forum (WEF), a group of senior people from the pharmaceutical industry, foundations and politicians including Børge Brende gathered for a brief meeting. In this elevated arena, Godal and his ideas benefited from having the backing of the Norwegian government. Norway benefited from being a wealthy and generous country, described by Chris Elias, president of the Global Health Division of the Gates Foundation as a 'thought leader' in global health problem solving.[89] Being one of the first countries to promote the idea of 'health security' locating health in a broader strategic context, and having shown leadership on Ebola, the decision was made at Davos, proposed by Jeremy Farrar, that the interim secretariat should be established in Norway, while the WEF should remain in close touch with developments to translate a concept into a practical organisation. The meeting agreed to aim for an ambitious official launch date of the new entity at the next WEF meeting in January 2017, and in the meantime, there would be a small interim secretariat overseeing a Working Group from all sectors of the assemblage.[90] John-Arne Røttingen became leader of the secretariat, and Godal, an influential member of the Working Group. Operating under the strictures of a non-negotiable timetable, three expert Task Teams ironed out many of the technical issues that threatened to frustrate the formation of their rapid-response organisation. In the months leading up to a workshop held in Oslo in April, they succeeded in designing the template for a new global non-profit multilateral start-up, which would work with existing organisations, that was entrepreneurial, and that had pharmaceutical companies baked into the governance although knowing that this might make some members of the organisation understandably paranoid.[91]

One of the influential pharma executives attending those meetings was Swati Gupta, executive director of Merck's office of Public Health and Science, and her experiences speaks to the reality and the indelible birth pangs of an entity advocating a more coordinated approach to vaccine development and pandemic response.

> Those meetings were very exciting because we knew that something great was happening, and everybody was very enthusiastic about making it happen. Sometimes you left and you felt a bit deflated because you knew it was going to be hard, and other times you would be uplifted because you could feel the needle moving finally towards the formation of this organisation.[92]

Mark Feinberg was another member of the Interim Coordinating Group and saw at first hand Godal's work behind the scenes, cajoling, coaxing and persuading others to strive for an agreement.

> Tore has a lot of great foresight. He is a quiet person, and I think I understand him, but it took me a long while. . . . When I first met him, I did not appreciate how influential he can be. But, he is; and his championing of CEPI was decisive in making it happen. I do not think CEPI would exist without Tore. That history is not so different from GAVI, where he had a vision and played an important role bringing together and encouraging other stakeholders to go after what had not been effectively addressed previously.[93]

One month later, on Wednesday, 17 May, a large follow-up conference took place at the National Academy of Sciences, on Constitution Avenue, Washington, DC. As the day wore on, Godal could sense a growing air of equivocation, what he describes as the 'wheels starting to spin as we were going over the same issues that we had discussed in Oslo a month earlier'.[94] More worryingly, some people raised the issue of whether they had the necessary mandate to develop an initiative! In a building known as the 'Temple of Science', Godal met these reservations with an assurance that he had never been involved in something with a stronger mandate. He sought to disabuse people by pointing out that there had been four independent reviews, including one established by the UN Secretary-General, and all four had recommended an intensified effort to develop new vaccines, and identified the lack of preparation as the major problem against pandemics. Standing shoulder-to-shoulder with Godal was Jeremy Farrar, the deep-thinking and dynamic Director of the Wellcome Trust.

> I gave a talk and argued if not 'us' then who? Who had a mandate? It was for those who could, to act, to be transparent, to gain as much support as possible, but if everyone waited for a mandate it would be too late – and who would that mandate come from anyway?[95]

This wise counsel proved persuasive, but the new organisation was proving to be an 'immensely complex beast',[96] and there was a pervasive sense of uncertainty as to how to move forward. It was a propitious moment, as Godal sensed the creation of what he and many others wanted, principally *a formal structured initiative*, would not carry the day, because some saw it as being too big a jump to make. Remembering the lessons from his own history, Godal recalled that almost two decades before, while planning the formulation of GAVI, the Vaccine Alliance, he had been able to circumvent similar objections by forming an intermediate agency: an *interim* organisation. This temporary plan outlined by Godal was both courageous and perilous, but it restored confidence, bridged a conceptual gulf, and the interim template became the casebook nexus and manifesto for CEPI.

On 20 May, when Godal returned to Oslo, he wrote a one-page outline, titled *Plan for Accelerated Development of CEPI*, of how the group could appoint an interim CEO by the end of June, an interim scientific advisory committee by the end of July, and an interim Board by the middle of August. He then sent the document to Jeremy Farrar, John-Arne Røttingen and Peter Piot, who duly approved his strategy:

Plan for Accelerated Development of CEPI

- Define 2016 and 2017 as start-up phase.
- Appoint interim CEO and Secretariat for the start-up phase by 17 June.
- Seek nominations to Board and Scientific Committee by 10 June.
- Establish interim Board and Scientific and Advisory Committee by 1 August.
- First meeting of Scientific Committee 1 September.
- First meeting by Board 2 September.
- First round of soliciting proposals Full or 'letters of intent' 5 September.
- Deadline 20 October. Review by Advisory group.
- Second Board meeting in India 10 November.
- Launch January WEF at Davos.[97]

Godal's proficiency was in designing, envisaging and establishing global health programmes and then stepping back to allow others to develop and grow the concept. In the summer of 2016, he believed that the obvious candidate for the interim CEO position was his protégé John-Arne Røttingen. Alas, like many of the best-laid plans, in early June, Røttingen announced that he had accepted the prestigious position of CEO of the Research Council of Norway (RCN). Over the summer, Godal tried in vain to persuade Røttingen that the CEPI appointment would be more rewarding; however, he did convince him to postpone his RCN role for nine months, thereby allowing time to navigate the politically delicate manoeuvring leading up to the launch in 2017. A pivotal moment in the launch timetable occurred in early September when the interim Board met for the first time at the Wellcome Trust headquarters in London. The meeting, chaired by Krishnaswamy VijayRaghavan, established an interim structure, an advanced business plan and finally, after almost a year, their organisation had a formal name, the 'Coalition for Epidemic Preparedness Innovation' (CEPI for short, pronounced 'Seppy').[98] Everything was now in place, and CEPI could turn its full attention to the serious business of fundraising the hundreds of millions of dollars it would need for the official launch in Davos in January 2017. To that end, the Core Group envisioned a model combining state and private funding under the umbrella of a comprehensive financing facility. Sophisticated charm offensives were set in motion targeting individual countries, and international conferences. To this end, at the G20 meeting, held on 4–5 September 2016, in the Chinese city of Hangzhou, the special guest speaker was the Norwegian Prime Minister, Erna Solberg who used the opportunity to speak on global public health. During her address, Erna Solberg announced that the Norwegian government would donate an additional US$75 million to CEPI. Behind the scenes, Godal was working away feverishly solidifying his links with Australia, India and Germany; meanwhile, his colleagues Jeremy Farrar and John-Arne Røttingen were turning their collective attentions to Japan.

Just a few days after the first CEPI Board meeting in London, on 11–12 September, Jeremy Farrar and John-Arne Røttingen attended the G7 Health Ministers' Meeting in Kobe, Japan, hosted by Shiozaki Yasuhisa, Minister of Health, Labour and Welfare, Japan. They were both determined to show the importance of CEPI to Japan in terms of biosecurity, innovation and global public health. The logic of their approach owed much to the enthusiasm shown by the world leaders of the G7 summit, which took place in May in the city of Shima, Japan. There the political elite stressed the importance of strengthening the response to widespread epidemics by taking into account the lessons learned from previous outbreaks like the Ebola virus epidemic in West Africa. Jeremy Farrar and John-Arne Røttingen sought to harness this powerful discourse on health and translate it into concrete financial and political support for CEPI. For their part, Japanese officials wanted to become involved in shaping the new endeavour and having their own pharmaceutical industry play a role in the multilateral collaboration. During the negotiations, it became clear that the role of Norway as an

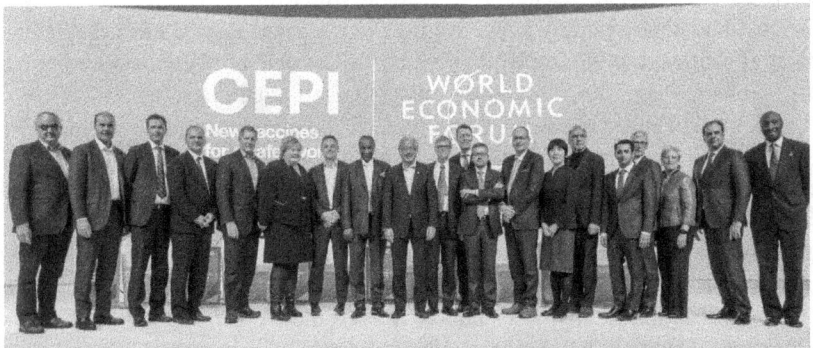

Figure 6.1 Luminaries from the world of politics, academia, medicine, industry and philanthropy, including among others Seth Berkley, Jeremy Farrar, Erna Solberg, Bill Gates, Peter Piot and John-Arne Røttingen came together for the formal launch of the Coalition for Epidemic Preparedness Innovations (CEPI) at the World Economic Forum at Davos, 2017.

Source: Courtesy of Frederik Kristensen/CEPI.

independent arbiter was critical in aligning the political and financial power of Japan to CEPI. Up until the autumn of 2016, the Japanese Ministry of Health was suspicious that CEPI with its UK, French and the US involvement may have a hidden agenda – to promote the donor country's vaccine industry. This would have been damaging to Japan; as like many other countries, they wanted to support their own vaccine industry as an important facet of health security. At the Kobe conference, John-Arne Røttingen became aware of the indispensability of Norway to CEPI's legitimacy when he met with Naoko Yamamoto, assistant Minister for Global Health, Labour and Welfare. From his Japanese colleague he learned that because Norway did not have a big pharmaceutical industry of its own, this removed any semblance of partisanship. Indeed, Naoko Yamamoto went on to describe how Japan admired Norway's global health leadership for being, 'open, neutral' and 'fair'.[99] When John-Arne Røttingen offered Japan a seat on the Interim Board of CEPI, he was confident that their relationship would bring future funding commitments from the Ministry of Health. 'We will only do this', Naoko Yamamoto said, 'because Norway is leading it, and as long as CEPI is a global neutral organisation that gives everyone a chance to contribute'.[100] In parallel, on the other side of the world, Godal was deploying the soft arts of persuasion on the German government in choreographed diplomacy with the Norwegian Ministry of Foreign Affairs.

Godal was in close contact with Mathias Licharz, inside the office of the German Chancellor, Angela Merkel. Licharz was responsible for development affairs and would later become Germany's ambassador to the UN Security Council. Godal and Licharz had established a good working relationship two years earlier when Angela Merkel and Erna Solberg were involved in the UN Secretary-General's purview of the Ebola outbreak.[101] Seen as a trusted global ambassador for health, Marhias Licharz introduced Godal to Joachim Klein in the Ministry of Education and Research indicating that they had, 'resources to invest'.[102] Having spent many decades at the epicentre of global health thinking, Godal had succeeded in showing how Norway's wise investment in health could yield immense results in terms of reduced child mortality, life improvement for adults and vast economic benefits for families and nations alike. Global health in turn was tremendously important for Norway because it delivers channels of diplomatic contact on other agendas. Both directly and indirectly, Godal managed to deliver Norwegian politicians international platforms where they had the opportunity to demonstrate leadership. Quite simply Godal understands the logic of politics, and he was able to identify the opportunities for partnerships to flourish. 'Germany and Japan were both very supportive', Borge Brende, the Norwegian Foreign Minister reminisced about the level of funding invested in the launch of CEPI, 'Tore did a lot of good ground work, I was just able to pick the apple'.[103]

As a counterpoint to the exhaustive development of complete business models, and highly sophisticated coordination mechanisms between different funders, when the leadership groups started formalising the institutional structure leading up to the January 2017 launch, they cultivated a policy of deliberate procedural opacity. The two principal architects of the policy of occasional inexactitude were Peter Piot and Godal. This was because in the final months of 2016 their primary objective was to preserve CEPI's momentum, and not to become diverted with hard and fast precedents, which would create endless debate, much soul-searching and unwanted delay. 'So, you need some tricks', is how Peter Piot diplomatically described their tactics of obfuscation.

> Tore and I had to improvise and it is as much an art as it is a science. . . . When we discussed the number of Board members, what kind of people, how many seats, frankly [it was] a kind of horse-trading, but that is what we did. Sometimes a lack of clarity is not so bad. We were pragmatic. But, occasionally, at the end of a discussion with Tore, I would go home and say to myself, 'what the hell did we actually agree?'

Where no doubt or confusion existed, however, was the seriousness of the treat that a pandemic posed to global public health. In less than 20 years, there had been the SARS virus outbreak in 2002, followed by bird flu, then swine flu, Zika virus, Chikungunya, MERS and finally Ebola. The challenge for CEPI would be to invest in platform technologies that could be rapidly adapted to new and unknown pathogens, and reduce the time required for vaccine development, to prevent a local disease outbreak becoming a pandemic.

The difficulty faced by Godal and his colleagues who were trying desperately to raise money to stimulate, finance and coordinate vaccine development against diseases with epidemic potential[104] was that vast sums were being syphoned off into military and nuclear defence, while investment in pandemic preparation was merely a drop in the ocean by comparison. In his long history of raising money for global health ventures, Godal had learned that timing, and the presentation of 'the ask'[105] was everything. Notwithstanding the ethical dimension, the laws of actuarial science and cause-and-effect relationships were powerful factors determining allocation of resources for health for national governments and philanthropic institutions. Godal understood this reality more than most and never lost sight of finding innovative ways to provide the most cost-effective health care to the world's poorest people. Objective indicators, and measurable impact on people's lives, were the metrics used by Godal to articulate health as an investment and not simply as expenditure. He used this understandable logic to mobilise support for CEPI from the governments of Norway, Germany and Japan and from the world's wealthiest philanthropic agency, the Gates Foundation. The impact and effectiveness of Godal's campaigns, in relation to malaria control, immunisation and vaccines, made his ideas morally and economically persuasive to Chris Elias, the president of Global Development at the foundation.

Tore has been at the start of so many important initiatives at the foundation, and we often say 'GAVI was one of our first, largest, and best investments'. At the beginning of GAVI, the foundation made an unprecedented $750 million commitment and GAVI is still our largest single investment over twenty some years now. I forget the specific figure, but it is somewhere north of $300 million a year. So, if you add it up, Tore has been an expensive friend.[106]

The Gates Foundation went on to commit US$100 million to CEPI, and the Wellcome Trust contributed the same amount.

In the weeks leading up to the launch, there had been much debate about the selection of diseases that CEPI should prioritise.[107] Everyone on the Scientific Advisory Board, including the chair, Mark Feinberg, knew that the biggest threat was from Disease X, caused by a pathogen not previously designated in the scientific literature.[108] Meanwhile, there were calls for CEPI to develop a universal flu vaccine, but with the pharmaceutical industry already ploughing hundreds of millions of dollars annually into flu vaccine research; it was felt that if CEPI joined that venture, it would rapidly exhaust its comparatively limited resources. It is salient to remember that we still do not have a universal flu vaccine and the wait may be a long one.

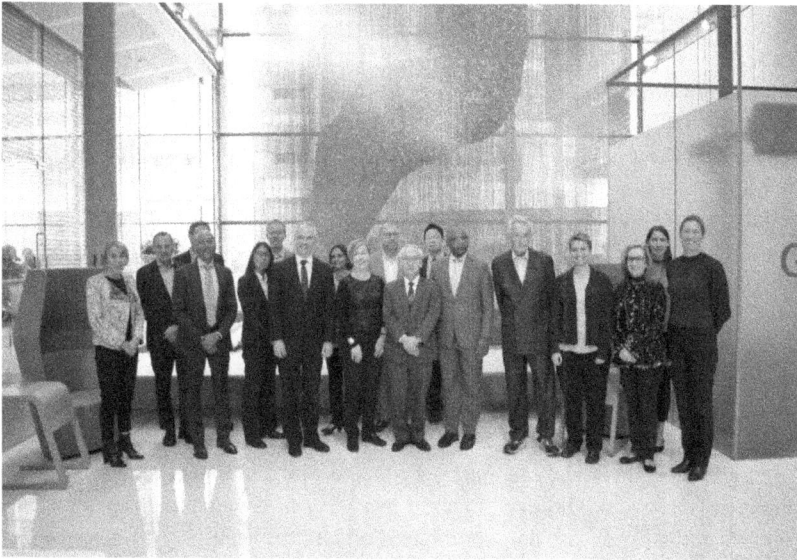

Figure 6.2 CEPI board meeting at the Wellcome Trust, London, October 2018. Tore Godal is fifth from the right. The photograph marked his final involvement as a member of the CEPI board.

Source: Courtesy of Frederik Kristensen/CEPI.

After a remarkably short gestation period of just 15 months, on 19 January 2017, the World Economic Forum launched the Coalition for Epidemic Preparedness Innovations (CEPI) in Davos. The public–private coalition received multi-year funding from Norway, Japan, Germany, the Bill and Melinda Gates Foundation and the Wellcome Trust, totalling US$545 million. In record time, soft promises had been turned into hard donations, and $545 million was, to the fiduciary-minded Godal, 'sufficient for the programme to start'.[109] That evening, CEPI made a first call for candidate vaccines against Lassa virus, Middle East Respiratory Syndrome coronavirus (MERS-CoV) and Nipah virus. The launch of CEPI, for Seth Berkley, CEO of GAVI, with 'the steady hand of Tore fathering the development',[110] showed that the Ebola outbreak had been a turning point and that the new coalition was a valuable contribution to ensuring the world has the vaccines it needs before epidemics begin.

CEPI is a Norwegian Association and is something of an anomaly in global public health, in that its Secretariat and headquarters are in Oslo, and not in Geneva, the Silicone Valley of world health governance. Rather than being viewed by Norwegians as some type of national trophy, its geographical setting is more of an acknowledgement of Norway's importance in the ecosystem of global public health and a recognition that not everything has to be located in Switzerland.[111]

At the end of February 2018, John-Arne Røttingen relinquished his caretaker role of CEO of CEPI and the US physician Richard Hatchett, a former White House adviser during the H1N1 outbreak of 2009, took up the position. Hatchett was an ideal appointment; he understood vaccinology and was highly experienced having led medical counter measure programmes at the Biomedical Advanced Research and Development Authority (BARDA) in the United States, including planning for responding to the Ebola, MERS and Zika outbreaks.[112] Godal's role as the builder of a missing piece in the global health architecture was now ending. Once he was sure that CEPI was firmly established, he contacted his friend, skiing partner and renowned international civil servant, Jane Halton, and asked her to Chair the Coalition. Jane Halton was highly respected in the hierarchies of power in Geneva, and as a former Secretary of the Australian Department of Finance, Godal had confidence that his friend would act as protection against the dark arts of political and non-evidence-based interference that CEPI might later encounter. When Godal stepped down from the Board at the end of 2018, he knew that another pandemic was imminent and that CEPI's long-term survival would depend upon its ability to develop and then distribute vaccines equitably across the world based on clinical need.

Notes

1. This epigram related to the Eastern Congo Ebola outbreak (2018–2020), which is the second-biggest ever 3,000 cases, as against 30,000 in the West Africa outbreak.

2. Sir Richard Peto, email communication February 2020. In 2021, there was another outbreak of Ebola in Guinea, infecting at least 18 people and killing nine by the middle of March. Close examination of the virus showed it be almost identical to the strain that caused the earlier outbreak. On this occasion, vaccinations, using the ring vaccination method began quickly.

3. A. Rojek, P. Horby, J. Dunning, "Insights from clinical research completed during the west African Ebola virus disease epidemic", *Lancet Infect Dis*, 2017, 17, pp. 280–292.

4. National Academies of Sciences, Engineer, and Medicine, *Integrating Clinical Research Into Epidemic Response: The Ebola Experience* (Washington, DC: The National Academies Press, 2017).

5. A. Rojek, P. W. Horby, "Offering patients more: How the West Africa Ebola outbreak can shape innovation in therapeutic research for emerging and epidemic infections", *Philosophical Transactions of the Royal Society of London. Series B, Biological Sciences*, 2017, 372, p. 20160294.

6. Interview with Tore Godal, August 2018.

7. M. B. A. Oldstone, *Viruses, Plagues, & History: Past Present and Future* (Oxford: Oxford University Press, 2010), p. 214.

8. M. B. A. Oldstone, *Viruses, Plagues, & History: Past Present and Future* (Oxford: Oxford University Press, 2010), p. 220.

9. P. B. Medawar, J. S. Medawar, *Aristotle to Zoos: A Philosophical Dictionary of Biology* (Cambridge: Cambridge University Press, 1983).

10. National Academies of Science, Engineering, and Medicine, *Integrating Clinical Research Into Epidemic Response: The Ebola Experience* (Washington, DC: The National Academies Press, 2017).

11. Interview with Ripley Ballou, September 2021.

12. Okairos specialised in making vaccines that target the immune systems' CD8 T cells, an approach that could lead to preventable vaccines against several infectious diseases. Tellingly, those who recovered from Ebola display an antiviral CD8 T cell response and antiviral antibody response.

13. Interview with Ripley Ballou, September 2021.

14. M. P. Kieny, "From vaccines to global health vaccines", *Human Vaccines and Immunotherapeutics Journal*, 2018, pp. 2550–2552.

15. Interview with Marie-Paule Kieny, October 2021.

16. GHRF Commission (Commission on a Global Health Risk Framework for the Future), *The neglected dimension of global security: A framework to counter infectious disease crisis.*

17. Interview with Marie-Paule Kieny, October 2021.

18. WHO, "Ebola R&D landscape of clinical candidates and trials", October 2015.

19. WHO, *Ethical Considerations for Use of Unregistered Interventions for Ebola virus Disease* (Geneva: WHO, 2014).

20. National Academies of Science, Engineering, and Medicine, *Integrating Clinical Research Into Epidemic Response: The Ebola Experience* (Washington, DC: The National Academies Press, 2017).

21. B. Ki-moon, *Resolved Uniting Nations in a Divided World* (New York: Columbia University Press, 2021), p. 238.

22. National Academies of Science, Engineering, and Medicine, *Integrating Clinical Research Into Epidemic Response: The Ebola Experience* (Washington, DC: The National Academies Press, 2017).

23. T. Mooney, E. Smout, E. Leigh, B. Greenwood, L. Enria, D. Ishola, D. Manno, M. Samai, M. Douoguih, D. Watson-Jones, "EBOVAC-salone: Lessons learned from

implementing an Ebola vaccine trial in an Ebola-affected country", *Clinical Trials*, 2018, 15 (5), pp. 436–443.

24. Jeremy Farrar believes that 'if you don't know something then I think it is unethical not to conduct a study, but RCTs don't exist in a vacuum, they exist in the context of the community they are happening in'.

25. C. Keating, *Smoking Kills: The Revolutionary Life of Richard Doll* (Oxford: Signal Books, 2009), p. 68.

26. Interview with Marie-Paule Kieny, October 2021.

27. National Academies of Science, Engineering, and Medicine, *Integrating Clinical Research Into Epidemic Response: The Ebola Experience* (Washington, DC: The National Academies Press, 2017).

28. C. Keating, *Smoking Kills: The Revolutionary Life of Richard Doll* (Oxford: Signal Books, 2009), p. 91.

29. National Academies of Science, Engineering, and Medicine, *Integrating Clinical Research Into Epidemic Response: The Ebola Experience* (Washington, DC: The National Academies Press, 2017).

30. Interview with Marie-Paule Kieny, October 2021.

31. Interview with John-Arne Røttingen, November 2019.

32. Godal saw it in terms of "David against Goliath".

33. Interview with Tore Godal, August 2021.

34. A. de Bengy Puyvallée, "Securitization of a humanitarian crisis: *Norway's International response to Ebola*", Master thesis in Culture, Environment and Sustainability, University of Oslo, Reprosentralen, 2017, p. 23.

35. Interview with Jeremy Farrar, August 2018.

36. Interview with Marie-Paule Kieny, October 2021.

37. S. B. Gupta, B. A. Coller, M. Feinberg, "Unprecedented pace of partnerships: The story of lessons learned from one Ebola vaccine program", *Expert Review Vaccines*, 2008, p. 2.

38. Interview with Tore Godal, August 2021.

39. Interview with Marie-Paule Kieny, October 2021.

40. In Guinea, two trials ran in parallel – the Ring Vaccination Trial and a phase II front-line worker safety and immunogenicity study in approximately 2,800 participants.

41. S. B. Gupta, B. A. Coller, M. Feinberg, "Unprecedented pace of partnerships: The story of lessons learned from one Ebola vaccine program", *Expert Review Vaccines*, 2008, p. 3.

42. Interview with John-Arne Røttingen, November 2019.

43. Interview with John-Arne Røttingen, November 2019.

44. Interview with Marie-Paule Kieny, October 2021.

45. Interview with Swati Gupta, November 2021.

46. S. Gilbert, C. Green, *Vaxxers: The Inside Story of the Oxford AstraZeneca Vaccine and the Race Against the Virus* (London: Hodder & Stoughton, 2021), p. 45.

47. A. Rojek, P. Horby, J. Dunning, "Insights from clinical research completed during the west African Ebola virus disease epidemic", *Lancet Infectious Diseases*, 2017, 17, p. e287.

48. A. M. Henao-Restrepo, I. M. Longin, M. Egger et al., "Efficacy and effectiveness of an rVSV-vectored vaccine expressing Ebola surface glycoprotein: Interim results from the Guinea ring vaccination cluster-randomised trial", *Lancet*, 2015, 386, pp. 857–866.

49. National Academies of Science, Engineering, and Medicine, *Integrating Clinical Research Into Epidemic Response: The Ebola Experience* (Washington, DC: The National Academies Press, 2017).

50. S. Prideaux, *I Am Dynamite! The Life of Friedrich Nietzsche* (London: Faber & Faber, 2018), p. 389.
51. Interview with Marie-Paule Kieny, October 2021.
52. National Academies of Science, Engineering, and Medicine, *Integrating Clinical Research Into Epidemic Response: The Ebola Experience* (Washington, DC: The National Academies Press, 2017).
53. A. Rid, F. G. Miller, "Ethical rational for the Ebola 'ring vaccination' trial design", *American Journal of Public Health*, 2016, 106 (3), pp. 432–435.
54. Thomas M. Burton in the Wall Street Journal 11 October 2017 wrote that a detailed report by the prestigious National Academy of Medicine in April questioned the methodology of the Merck vaccine study in Guinea. It concluded the Merck vaccine 'most likely provides some protections', to recipients but that the protection 'could in reality be low'. In another article written by Thomas M. Burton, John-Arne Røttingen felt that his comments had not been quoted in full, and that Cliff Lane of the National Institute of the Allergy and Infectious Diseases (NIAID) had said the trial treated people as 'guinea pigs'. However, when John-Arne Røttingen met with Tony Fauci, the Director of NIAID, he told John-Arne that he was pleased with the Ebola trial and offered his congratulations.
55. Interview with Marie-Paule Kieny, October 2021.
56. Interview with John-Arne Røttingen, November 2019.
57. Interview with Mark Feinberg, November 2021.
58. Interview with Ripley Ballou, September 2021.
59. S. Gilbert, C. Green, *Vaxxers: The Inside Story of the Oxford AstraZeneca Vaccine and the Race Against the Virus* (London: Hodder & Stoughton, 2021), p. 41.
60. S. Gilbert, C. Green, *Vaxxers: The Inside Story of the Oxford AstraZeneca Vaccine and the Race Against the Virus* (London: Hodder & Stoughton, 2021), p. 47.
61. GHRF (Commission on a Global Health Framework for the Future), *The Neglected Dimension of Global Security: A Framework to Counter Infectious Disease Crises* (2016), p. 4.
62. Interview with Ripley Ballou, September 2021.
63. Interview with Marie-Paule Kieny, October 2021.
64. Interview with Seth Berkley, November 2019.
65. S. Moon, D. Sridhar, M. A. Pate, A. K. Jha, C. Clinton, S. Delaunay, V. Edwin, M. Fallah, D. P. Fidler, L. Garrett, E. Goosby, L. O. Gostin, D. L. Heymann, K. Lee, G. M. Leung, J. S. Morrison, J. Saavedra, M. Tanner, J. A. Leigh, B. Hawkins, L. R. Woskie, P. Piot, "Will Ebola change the game? Ten essential reforms before the next pandemic: The report of the Harvard-LSHTM independent panel on the global response to Ebola", *Lancet*, 28 November 2015, 386 (10009), pp. 2204–2221.
66. S. A. Plotkin, A. A. Mahmoud, J. Farrar, "Establishing a global vaccine-development fund", *New England Journal of Medicine*, 2015, 373 (4), pp. 297–300.
67. S. A. Plotkin, A. A. Mahmoud, J. Farrar, "Establishing a global vaccine-development fund", *New England Journal of Medicine*, 2015, 373 (4), pp. 297–300.
68. Interview with Tore Godal, November 2019.
69. H. D. Klenk, S. Becker, "Ebola virus vaccines – preparing for the unexpected", *Science*, 2015, 349 (6249), pp. 693–694.
70. Interview with Tore Godal, November 2019.
71. Interview with Børge Brende, November 2021.
72. A. de Bengy Puyvallée, "Securitization of a humanitarian crisis: *Norway's International Response to Ebola*", Master thesis in Culture, Environment and Sustainability, University of Oslo, Reprosentralen, 2017, p. III.
73. Interview with Helga Fogstad, June 2020.

74. Interview with Peter Piot, November 2021.
75. S. Moon, D. Sridhar, M. A. Pate, A. K. Jha, C. Clinton, S. Delaunay, V. Edwin, M. Fallah, D. P. Fidler, L. Garrett, E. Goosby, L. O. Gostin, D. L. Heymann, K. Lee, G. M. Leung, J. S. Morrison, J. Saavedra, M. Tanner, J. A. Leigh, B. Hawkins, L. R. Woskie, P. Piot, "Will Ebola change the game? Ten essential reforms before the next pandemic: The report of the Harvard-LSHTM independent panel on the global response to Ebola", *Lancet*, 2015, 386 (10009), pp. 2204–2221.
76. S. Moon, D. Sridhar, M. A. Pate, A. K. Jha, C. Clinton, S. Delaunay, V. Edwin, M. Fallah, D. P. Fidler, L. Garrett, E. Goosby, L. O. Gostin, D. L. Heymann, K. Lee, G. M. Leung, J. S. Morrison, J. Saavedra, M. Tanner, J. A. Leigh, B. Hawkins, L. R. Woskie, P. Piot, "Will Ebola change the game? Ten essential reforms before the next pandemic: The report of the Harvard-LSHTM independent panel on the global response to Ebola", *Lancet*, (2015), 386 (10009), pp. 2204–2221.
77. S. Moon, D. Sridhar, M. A. Pate, A. K. Jha, C. Clinton, S. Delaunay, V. Edwin, M. Fallah, D. P. Fidler, L. Garrett, E. Goosby, L. O. Gostin, D. L. Heymann, K. Lee, G. M. Leung, J. S. Morrison, J. Saavedra, M. Tanner, J. A. Leigh, B. Hawkins, L. R. Woskie, P. Piot, "Will Ebola change the game? Ten essential reforms before the next pandemic: The report of the Harvard-LSHTM independent panel on the global response to Ebola", *Lancet*, 2015, 386 (10009), pp. 2204–2221.
78. Interview with Peter Piot, November 2021.
79. D. L. Heymann, L. Chen, K. Takemi, D. P. Fidler, J. W. Tappero, M. J. Thomas, T. A. Kenyon, T. R. Frieden, D. Yach, S. Nishtar, A. Kalache, P. L. Olliaro, P. Horby, E. Torreele, L. O. Gostin, M. Ndomondo-Sigonda, D. Carpenter, S. Rushton, L. Lillywhite, B. Devkota, K. Koser, R. Yates, R. S. Dhillon, R. P. Rannan-Eliya, "Global health security: the wider lessons from the west African Ebola virus disease epidemic", *Lancet*, 2015, 385, pp. 1884–1901, 1885.
80. *An R&D Blueprint for Action to Prevent Epidemics: Plan of Action* (Geneva: WHO Document Production Services, 2016).
81. Interview with Marie-Paule Kieny, October 2021.
82. I. K. Sandberg, S. Andresen, U. Gopinathan, B. S. Hustad Hembre, "The formation of the Coalition for Epidemic Preparedness Innovations (CEPI): An empirical study", *Wellcome Open Research*, 2020, 5, p. 284.
83. Interview with Jeremy Farrar, August 2018.
84. Interview with Jeremy Farrar, August 2018.
85. Interview with Peter Piot, November 2021.
86. Interview with Jeremy Farrar, August 2018.
87. Interview with Jeremy Farrar, August 2018.
88. Interview with John-Arne Røttingen, November 2019.
89. Interview with Chris Elias, December 2021.
90. I. K. Sandberg, S. Andresen, U. Gopinathan, B. S. Hustad Hembre, "The formation of the Coalition for Epidemic Preparedness Innovations (CEPI): An empirical study", *Wellcome Open Res*, 2020, 5, p. 284.
91. Interview with Peter Piot, November 2021.
92. Interview with Swati Gupta, November 2021.
93. Interview with Mark Feinberg, November 2021.
94. Interview with Tore Godal, August 2018.
95. Personal communication, email Jeremy Farrar, December 2021.
96. Interview with Jeremy Farrar, August 2018.
97. Tore Godal, personal papers.
98. The CEPI mission emerged during these early discussions. 'We want to stop future epidemics by developing new vaccines for a safer world. Vaccines are one of the

world's most important health achievements, but their life-saving potential hasn't yet been realised by many known and unknown epidemic threats'.

99. Personal communication, email Naoko Yamamoto, December 2021.
100. Personal communication, email Naoko Yamamoto, December 2021.
101. The Secretary-General subsequently appointed Jakaya Mrisho Kikwete, President of the United Republic of Tanzania, as Chair.
102. Interview with Tore Godal, August 2018.
103. Interview with Borge Brende, November 2021.
104. S. B. Gupta, B. A. Coller, M. Feinberg, "Unprecedented pace of partnerships: The story of lessons learned from one Ebola vaccine program", *Expert Review Vaccines*, 2008, p. 8.
105. Interview with Tore Godal, August 2018.
106. Interview with Chris Elias, December 2021.
107. Stanley Plotkin was a member of the scientific advisory board. 'There was a lot of emphasis on taking the WHO list, which I fought. I thought the WHO was a "wish list" and I felt that we should select targets that are feasible in order to achieve success. For example, there were no bacterial diseases on the WHO list, which I thought was a mistake. I fought unsuccessfully for the choice of Chikungunya'.
108. Interview with Mark Feinberg, November 2021.
109. Interview with Tore Godal, August 2018.
110. "From Gavi to CEPI: The transformation of global health in the 21st century", speech by Seth Berkley, Kings Medal Awards, Oslo, 23 November 2019.
111. Interview with Borge Brende, November 2021.
112. Stanley Plotkin describes BARDA as "essentially a semi-military version of CEPI".

Epilogue

Tore Godal is a giant of public health and one of its unsung heroes.

WHO Director-General, Tedros Adhanom Ghebreyesus

On a rainy November afternoon in 2019, Tore Godal found himself back in Gamle Festsal, one of the historic main halls of the University of Oslo, the exact location where he had defended his PhD thesis on a bright, green June morning in 1967, and where his journey in global health had begun. During the intervening 52 years, the field of global health had been transformed from a neglected area of human endeavour to one at the forefront of scientific research, international development and foreign policy. In recent years alone, funding has shot up from $5 billion in 2000 to over $35 billion 20 years later. This has contributed to unprecedented reductions in child mortality, life improvement for adults and vast economic benefits for families and nations alike. Godal had returned to his alma mater to receive a national honour, The Norwegian King's Medal of Merit, in recognition of a lifetime of achievement in immunisation and global health. As the rain gently fell outside Gamle Festsal, inside government ministers, medics, cultural luminaries and Godal's friends and family gathered to celebrate the achievements of 'a great scientist, a medical pioneer, and a global health leader'.[1] Tore Godal's lifelong adhesion to improving global public health had started at the Armauer Hansen Research Institute (AHRI) in Addis Ababa, Ethiopia in the 1970s, where he had used the insights of the 'new immunology' to elucidate mechanisms of disease and to develop new treatments for leprosy. As he looked around the packed auditorium he could see his mentor, the celebrated Norwegian immunologist Morten Harboe, who had both refereed his PhD thesis and preceded him as Director of AHRI. Also present, and which gave him much satisfaction, was Abebe Genetu Bayih, Director-General of the Institute today. Godal's experiences in Ethiopia initiated an extraordinarily productive career that brought together preventive medicine and basic science to reduce human suffering and increase life expectancy. It is not too much to say that millions of people are alive today because of the decisive contributions that Godal has made to the health of the global community.

DOI: 10.4324/9781003363859-8

As Director as the Special Programme for Research and Training in Tropical Diseases (TDR), Godal established new global partnerships and sponsored research into vaccines for leprosy and malaria; under his leadership, TDR has had a lasting influence on international science which had a multiplier effect, as young scientists realised the immense importance, fascination and potential of tropical disease research. During more than a decade in Geneva, Godal also made decisive contributions to the treatment of river blindness by sponsoring large randomised controlled trials of the anti-parasitic drug ivermectin, showing that the medication was both safe and that it could be distributed by community volunteers. However, the most devastating of all the infectious disease affecting populations in Africa is malaria, and in the 1990s, the disease killed one million people every year, mostly children. The decisive moment in the history of malaria control was Godal's funding of the large cluster randomised controlled trial of insecticide-treated bed nets on the mortality of Gambian children in the early 1990s. Today, insecticide bed nets form the cornerstone of malaria control programmes in Africa and beyond.

A similarly pivotal moment in the contemporary history of immunisation was when Godal established Gavi, the Vaccine Alliance in 2000. Since that date, the proportion of children globally receiving routine immunisation has risen from 60% to 86%, resulting in a 70% decline in vaccine-preventable disease mortality. Leading this new public–private entity through the difficult early years of its existence was only possible, according to one historian, because of the defining role played by Godal who acted 'as the glue that holds things together'.[2] The Millennium Development Goals (MDGs) marked another inflection point for global health innovation. As a systems thinker and innovator, Godal created a decisive moment in maternal and child welfare when he introduced performance-based financing into health care. By liberating development funds in the World Bank, Godal was able to champion MDGs 4 and 5, establishing the programmes *Every Woman Every Child* and *The Global Financing Facility*, and in due course, influencing the health of women and children across the globe. These programmes have been truly life changing: since 1990, under-five mortality has declined by over 50%, while global maternal death rates dropped by almost 40% in the same period.

The final decisive moment explored in this book was Godal's foundational work in creating, designing and financing the Coalition for Epidemic Preparedness Innovations (CEPI) in 2017, to ensure that the world would have vaccines against emerging infectious diseases, before epidemics and pandemics begin. Two other physician-scientists in attendance on that damp November day in Oslo were Seth Berkley, CEO of Gavi, The Vaccine Alliance and Richard Hatchett, CEO of CEPI. Both organisations owed their existence to the steady hand and visionary ideas of Godal, and even though he had persuaded the Norwegian Institute of Public Health to use the award ceremony as a platform for an Honorary Seminar titled *Global Health: Lessons for the Future of Priority Setting*, no-one in the room could have foreseen the devastation of the COVID-19 pandemic.

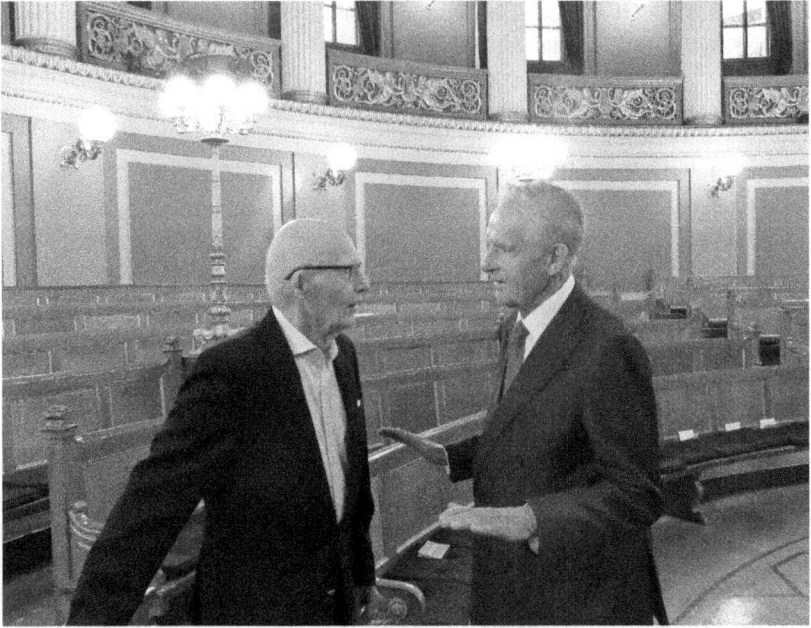

Figure 7.1 On 23 November 2019, Tore Godal received The King's Medal of Merit Award for his work in global health. It seemed only fitting that among the invited guests was his friend and mentor Morton Harboe: the men were once again reunited in Gamle Festsal, the room where Godal had defended his thesis in 1967, and where his long career in global health had begun.

Source: Courtesy of Andy Crump.

In only a matter of months, CEPI and GAVI, together with WHO and UNICEF would create COVAX as a vehicle to accelerate the development, production and equitable access to COVID-19 tests, treatments and vaccines across the world.

One of the speakers at the award ceremony was Norway's current Prime Minister, Jonas Gahr Støre, who used the occasion to praise his friend and to articulate a hypothesis that the twenty-first century had witnessed a great acceleration in global health in terms of innovation and demonstrable results.[3] By focusing his efforts on cost-effective investments directed at reducing mortality and bringing together assemblages of people who had not previously collaborated, Godal has made an important contribution to this acceleration, and more profoundly, to improving the conditions of human life. In fact, the great super-charging of global health innovation and investment corresponds with the remarkable Indian summer of Godal's career. Since his first 'enforced' retirement in 1999, Tore Godal has had a prodigious later career punctuated by episodic retirements and epoch-making transformational changes to the global health landscape. He has achieved so much by building a nexus of trust with collections of people across the world of politics and medical science, in the World Bank, WHO and philanthropic agencies, and has inspired them by his selflessness, moral authority, determination and the power of example. It is certainly true that one of the secrets to Godal's success has been that his loyalty was always to the global health mission in general, and not to a specific job or institution. To realise these bigger objectives, he needed to form allegiances with different groups. Throughout his working life, he persuaded people from varied organisations and governments to behave as if they were one team, even though they were very far from this in reality. His brand of leadership was to lead by example, under the mantra 'your word is your word, and that is it!'[4] Godal's role in these episodes, as mapped out in this volume, has been both undeniable and absolutely central. Yet these are not stories in which one individual's vision and will alone was the determining factor in transforming a field. As we have witnessed, these eclectic decisive moments sometimes revolve around ideas, strategies or inventions, while on other occasions they represent the power of people, institutions and collaboration. Godal's

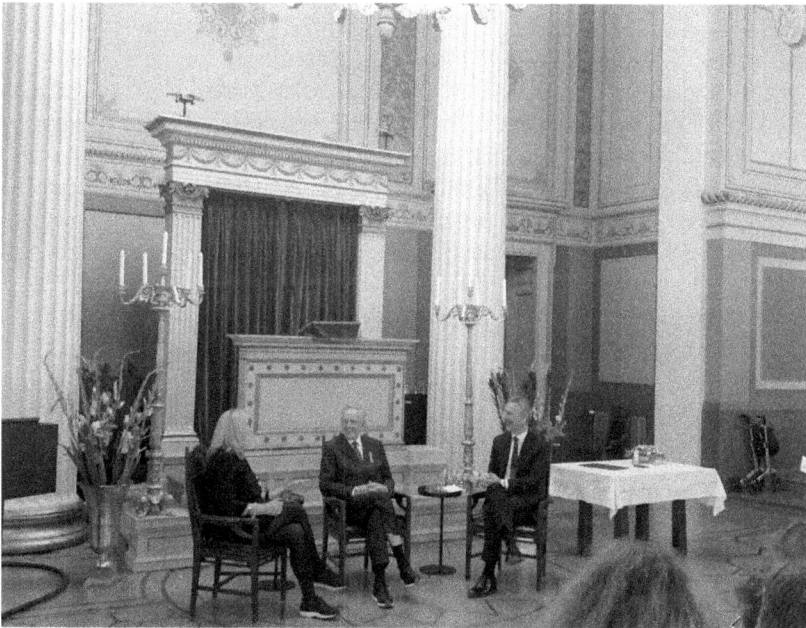

Figure 7.2 As part of the King's Medal of Merit award ceremony, Tore Godal and the former Norwegian Prime Minister Jens Stoltenberg discussed with the journalist Anne Grossvold their past initiatives in global vaccination and immunization, and lessons for the future of priority setting in global public health.

Source: Courtesy of Frederik Kristensen/CEPI.

presence in connecting each of these episodes tells us not simply about his own scientific and intellectual prowess but also of the value of creating networks of creative and ambitious researchers, politicians and philanthropists to tackle some of the biggest issues on the planet. While one man has disproportionately influenced the world of global health, the nature of his interventions once again demonstrate that global health is a collective rather than an individual pursuit.

Despite Godal's global role, his career rests on inherently local, personal values. Growing up in his valley home in the village of Rauland in rural Norway, he listened to both the moral and religious principles of his clergyman father, and his mother's ethereal fairy tales of audacity and daring.[5] It was there that he learned to become a proficient cross-country skier, and where he first thought about becoming a District Medical Officer serving the people in his native valley. That early dream would later transcend national boundaries, and over the decades through his work as a doctor, scientist, field worker and global health diplomat, Tore Godal has become the closest thing we have to the World's District Medical Officer. Perhaps, there is no disjunction between the mysticism of fairy tales and the materialism of science: global public health needs dreamers after all, people who want to help the world and change it for the better. Now in his 84th year, Godal continues to work full-time in his capacity as advisor to the Norwegian Ministry of Health and Care Services and as advisor to WHO Director-General, Tedros Adhanom Ghebreyesus. We are going to need more people like Tore Godal in the future. The challenges we face in the twenty-first century are fundamentally global, our world ever-more interconnected, as demonstrated so powerfully by the COVID-19 pandemic and the impending threat of climate change. Godal through his ability to seize, shape and influence decisive moments has helped to deliver sustainable, global health programmes that have increased life expectancy and reduced the burden of disease. His greatest legacy may well be to the values that define his character and by which he unselfishly lives: anonymity, public service and leadership.

Notes

1. S. Berkley, "From Gavi to CEPI: The transformation of global health in the 21st century", speech given on 23 November 2019.
2. W. Muraskin, *Crusade to Immunize the World's Children* (Los Angeles: Global Biobusiness Books: University of Southern California, 2005), p. 135.
3. J. Gahr Støre, "At the turn of the millennium, a new momentum for global health innovation: What made it happen?", speech given on 23rd November, 2019.
4. Interview with Tore Godal, November 2019.
5. C. Keating, *Kenneth Warren and the Great Neglected Diseases of Mankind: The Transformation of Geographical Medicine in the US and Beyond* (New York: Springer, 2017), p. 57.

Index

Note: Page numbers in *italics* indicate figures.

Taylor & Francis Group
an **informa** business

Taylor & Francis eBooks

www.taylorfrancis.com

A single destination for eBooks from Taylor & Francis
with increased functionality and an improved user
experience to meet the needs of our customers.

90,000+ eBooks of award-winning academic content in
Humanities, Social Science, Science, Technology, Engineering,
and Medical written by a global network of editors and authors.

TAYLOR & FRANCIS EBOOKS OFFERS:

A streamlined
experience for
our library
customers

A single point
of discovery
for all of our
eBook content

Improved
search and
discovery of
content at both
book and
chapter level

REQUEST A FREE TRIAL
support@taylorfrancis.com

Routledge
Taylor & Francis Group

CRC Press
Taylor & Francis Group

For Product Safety Concerns and Information please contact our EU
representative GPSR@taylorandfrancis.com
Taylor & Francis Verlag GmbH, Kaufingerstraße 24, 80331 München, Germany

www.ingramcontent.com/pod-product-compliance
Lightning Source LLC
Chambersburg PA
CBHW060259220326
41598CB00027B/4163